Clinical Otology

This volume is one of the series
Ear Clinics International
Michael M. Paparella and William L. Meyerhoff

Other books in this series include:

Paparella and Meyerhoff: Sensorineural Hearing Loss, Vertigo and
   Tinnitus
Paparella and Goycoolea: Clinical Problems In Otitis Media and
   Innovations in Surgical Otology

Ear Clinics International
VOLUME III

Clinical Otology

edited by
Michael M. Paparella, M.D.

Professor and Head
Department of Otolaryngology
University of Minnesota Medical School
Minneapolis, Minnesota
Director, Lions International Hearing Center

William L. Meyerhoff, M.D., Ph.D.

Professor and Chairman
Department of Otorhinolaryngology
University of Texas Health Science Center
Southwestern Medical School
Dallas, Texas

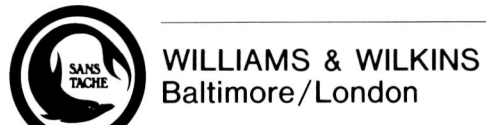

WILLIAMS & WILKINS
Baltimore/London

Copyright ©, 1983
Williams & Wilkins
428 East Preston Street
Baltimore, MD 21202, U.S.A.

All rights reserved. This book is protected by copyright. No part of this book may be reproduced in any form or by any means, including photocopying, or utilized by any information storage and retrieval system without written permission from the copyright owner.

Made in the United States of America

Library of Congress Cataloging in Publication Data

Main entry under title:

Clinical otology

(Ear clinics international; v. 3)
Includes index.
1. Ear—Diseases. 2. Ear—Surgery. I. Paparella, Michael M. II. Meyerhoff, William L. III. Series. [DNLM: 1. Ear diseases—Congresses. W3 EA117 v.3 1981 / WV 200 C641 1981]
RF121.C54   617.8   82-2603
ISBN 0-683-06748-6   AACR2

Composed and printed at the
Waverly Press, Inc.
Mt. Royal and Guilford Aves.
Baltimore, MD 21202, U.S.A.

Preface

This, the third volume of International Ear Clinics provides a blend of current concepts of ear problems and otological surgical considerations by expert Otologists from various countries.

In the "Otitis Media Surgery" section, early otitis media in childhood or otitis medial with effusion (OME) are discussed including considerations of pathogenesis, diagnosis, ventilation tubes, and tonsillectomy and adenoidectomy (Goycoolea, Bluestone, Meyerhoff) followed by a common sequella of otitis media-tympanosclerosis (Schiff). Then tempanoplasty and ossiculoplasty concepts are discussed (Fisch, Goodhill, Sheehy) with long-term results of cholesteatoma surgery and mastoid cavity care (Palva).

Current stapes surgery methods including stapedotomy by Fisch and stapedectomy revision by Sheehy reveal some new ideas in the surgical treatment of otosclerosis.

The application of auditory brain stem response as an aid in diagnosis (Harford and Harker) and clinical concepts of diagnosing acoustic tumors (Luetje) are presented after which middle ear cranial fossa surgical methods are discussed (Harker).

In the next section, some new and innovative concepts of diagnosis and treatment of labyrinthine problems are described including fistulas (Goodhill), sudden deafness (Schiff), autoimmune inner ear disease (McCabe), cochlear implants (Luetje), and tinnitus masking (Harford). These medical and surgical labyrinthine topics are new and, in some cases, too new to be established but time and experience will help define their respective roles in Otology.

The final section includes topics on vertigo and surgery for vertigo including classical methods of diagnosis and treatment (Jongkees), and current methods for using surgery to treat intractable vertigo (McCabe and Paparella).

As in other editions of International Ear Clinics, these international otological experts contribute to the continuing dialogue of evolving methods for diagnosing and treating otological problems. Rarely can any concept be considered "definitive", rather these discussions are dedicated to an ongoing search for truth.

Michael M. Paparella, M.D.

Contributors

Charles D. Bluestone, M.D.
Director, Department of Otolaryngology
Children's Hospital of Pittsburgh
Pittsburgh, PA

Ugo P. Fisch, M.D.
Professor of ENT
Head of Department of ENT
University of Zurich
University Hospital
Zurich, Switzerland

Victor Goodhill, M.D., F.A.C.S.
Adjunct Professor, Division of Head & Neck Surgery
UCLA Medical School
Los Angeles, CA

Marcos V. Goycoolea, M.D., M.S., Ph.D.
Instituto de Otologia y Cirugia de Cabez y Cuello
Santiago, Chile

Earl R. Harford, Ph.D.
Professor, Department of Otolaryngology
Director of Audiology
University of Minnesota School of Medicine
Minneapolis, MN

Lee A. Harker, M.D.
Professor, Department of Otolaryngology and Maxillofacial Surgery
University of Iowa Hospitals and Clinics
Iowa City, IA

Leonard B. W. Jongkees, Ph.D.
Professor, Head of Department of Otorhinololaryngology
University of Amsterdam
Amsterdam, Holland

Charles M. Luetje, M.D.
Assistant Clinical Professor
Department of Surgery
University of Missouri
Kansas City, Missouri

Brian McCabe
Professor & Head, Department of Otolaryngology & Maxillofacial Surgery
University of Iowa Hospitals & Clinics
Iowa City, IA

William L. Meyerhoff, M.D., Ph.D.
Professor and Chairman
Department of Otorhinolaryngology
Southwestern Medical School
Dallas, TX

Michael M. Paparella, M.D.
Professor & Head, Department of Otolaryngology
University of Minnesota School of Medicine
Minneapolis, MN

Tauno Palva, M.D.
Professor of Otolaryngology
Department of Otolaryngology
University of Helsinki
Helsinki, Finland

Maurice Schiff, M.D.
Clinical Professor
Department of Surgery
University of California, San Diego
San Diego, CA

James L. Sheehy, M.D.
Clinical Professor
Department of Otolaryngology
University of Southern California School of Medicine
Los Angeles, CA

Contents

Preface v

Contributors vii

Section I.
OTITIS MEDIA SURGERY

CHAPTER 1. **Pathogenesis of Otitis Media**
Marcos V. Goycoolea, M.D., M.S., Ph.D. 1

CHAPTER 2. **Efficacy of Various Methods of Therapy for Otitis Media**
Charles D. Bluestone, M.D. 3

CHAPTER 3. **Tympanostomy Tube Therapy for Otitis Media**
William L. Meyerhoff, M.D., Ph.D. 17

CHAPTER 4. **Status of Tonsillectomy and Adenoidectomy in the Treatment of Otitis Media**
Charles D. Bluestone, M.D. 21

CHAPTER 5. **Tympanosclerosis Cause and Prevention**
Maurice Schiff, M.D. 31

CHAPTER 6. **Cholesteatoma Surgery with Obliteration: Late Results**
Tauno Palva, M.D. 38

CHAPTER 7. **Total Reconstruction of the Ossicular Chain**
Ugo P. Fisch, M.D. 45

CHAPTER 8. **Prefabricated Allograft Ossiculoplasty**
Victor Goodhill, M.D. 52

CHAPTER 9. **Tympanoplasty: Postoperative Retraction Pockets and Residual Cholesteatoma**
James L. Sheehy, M.D. 68

CHAPTER 10. **Management of Open, Diseased Mastoid Cavity**
Tauno Palva, M.D. 73

Section II.
STAPES SURGERY

CHAPTER 11. **Stapedotomy versus Stapedectomy**
Ugo P. Fisch, M.D. 78

CHAPTER 12. **Experiences with Revision Stapedectomy**
James L. Sheehy, M.D. 85

Section III.
RETRO-COCHLEAR CONSIDERATION AND SURGERY

CHAPTER 13. **Variable Clinical Presentations of Acoustic Tumors**
Charles L. Luetje, M.D. 91

CHAPTER 14. **Middle Cranial Fossa Surgery**
Lee A. Harker, M.D. 101

CHAPTER 15. **Auditory Brain Stem Response (Short Latency)**
Earl R. Harford, Ph.D. 105

CHAPTER 16. **Auditory Brain Stem Response (Middle Latency)**
Lee A. Harker, M.D. 114

Section IV.
CURRENT CONCEPTS IN LABYRINTHINE DISEASE

CHAPTER 17. **Labyrinthine Fistulas**
Victor Goodhill, M.D. 118

CHAPTER 18. **A Sudden Hearing Loss**
Maurice Schiff, M.D. 128

CHAPTER 19. **Autoimmune Inner Ear Disease**
Brian McCabe, M.D. 137

CHAPTER 20. **Single Electrode Cochlear Implantation: A Coinvestigator Report**
Charles M. Luetje, M.D. 139

CHAPTER 21. **Tinnitus Masking: A Critical Review**
Earl R. Harford, Ph.D. 147

Section V.
VERTIGO AND SURGERY FOR VERTIGO

CHAPTER 22. **Ménière's Syndrome and Disease**
Leonard B. W. Jongkees, M.D. 151

CHAPTER 23. **Iowa Results of the Treatment of Ménière's Disease**
Brian F. McCabe, M.D. 153

CHAPTER 24. **Treatment of Vertigo**
Leonard B. W. Jongkees, M.D. 155

CHAPTER 25. **Critical Review of Endolympathic Sac Surgery**
Michael M. Paparella, M.D. 159

Index 165

CHAPTER 1
Pathogenesis of Otitis Media

Marcos V. Goycoolea, M.D., M.S., Ph.D.

Otitis media is an inflammatory disease of high incidence and prevalence which can evolve or resolve in a number of different and unpredictable manners. There are so many forms, complications, and/or sequelae that a general overview would necessarily end up as just a summary. It has been my purpose to describe our systematic approach to a single aspect, that is, subtle inner ear complications of otitis media. Since this is a review of our past and present experience, the literature will not be discussed. Complete discussions are included in our referenced papers.

Back in 1970, Drs. Paparella et al. (1) reported that otitis media could result not only in devastating inner ear changes such as suppurative labyrinthitis but also in subtle changes such as sensorineural hearing loss. Shortly thereafter, I came to Minnesota; we reviewed a large number of temporal bones with otitis media and observed that a significant number had the association of otitis media, round window membrane changes, and endolymphatic hydrops (2).

With this evidence in hand, we initiated a systematic experimental approach in order to verify or disprove these associations. The normal middle ear of the cat was described (3). The round window (light microscopy) appeared as a three-layered membrane with an outer epithelium (towards the middle ear) with a single layer of cuboidal cells, a middle core of connective tissue, and a flat squamous inner epithelium continuous with the one of the inner ear. The outer and middle layers are continuous with those of the middle ear, providing a continuity of blood and lymph vessels which are abundant at the lateral edges of the membrane.

Following this first step, a longitudinal study of histopathological changes in the middle ear of cats with induced otitis media (1 day to 6 months) was done (4). We observed that there are definite stages in the development of this disease, with definite patterns of cellular infiltration and effusion formation so we postulated the concept of a "Middle Ear Defense System" (5). Although this is not the main subject of this discussion, it must be mentioned that a clear understanding of this system is essential since it will eventually lead to a more rational and effective medical treatment of this disease. Hopefully, this could leave surgical procedures in an ideal role of restoration of function rather than that of erradication of disease.

From a general standpoint, if anything would pass from middle to inner ear it would do so necessarily via either the oval window, round window, bony fistulas, and/or blood or lymph vessels. With this in mind, we looked at the different areas in the middle ears of experimental animals and observed that in spite of all the changes, the oval window remained intact at all stages and that there were no bony fistulas (6). However, when we looked at the round window, it was evident that it followed the changes of the mucoperiosteum of the middle ear (7). The round window membrane changes were then quantified (8).

When we reviewed the literature, it was evident that the round window membrane, despite being three-layered, behaved like a semipermeable membrane. However, no studies had been done in permeability of macromolecules or toxins. In a group of animals with induced otitis media, we placed tritiated albumin in the round window niche and were able to recover it in perilymph 20 minutes later (9). We then placed tritiated staphylococcal exotoxin in the niche and recovered it in perilymph of both normal and otitis induced animals (10, 11). The question posed was no longer whether macromolecules or toxins could pass into the inner ear, but what happens when they get there. Based on these observations, we suggested the possibility of an "Inner Ear Defense System", since otherwise, the incidence of sensorineural hearing loss following otitis media would be extremely common. We used staphylococcal exotoxin because staph is a frequent organism in chronic otitis media, and these strains produce a large number of extracellular products, many of them potent toxins. Some of these toxins have the capability of not only injuring hair cells and nerve fibers but also of blocking sodium pumps. This becomes extremely interesting since there are diseases of the inner ear and inner fluid imbalances whose pathogenesis are not known.

At this point in time what was needed were ultrastructural studies that would provide more detailed information. So, upon my return to Chile, we initiated these studies with Anna-Mary Carpenter and David Muchow. An ultrastructural study of the cat round window membrane was done that revealed interesting features (12). The outer epithelium has extensive interdigitations between the cells and abundant tight junctions. The cells have sparse microvilli and abundant mitochondria as well as a well-developed Golgi. The basement membrane, thinner than that of the nearby promontory mucosa is continuous. The core of connective tissue is rich in blood and lymph vessels especially towards the edges. The inner epithelium has lining cells with long lateral extensions with sparse and inelaborate junctions. There is no continuous basement membrane. If we add our preliminary observations (unpublished) of pathological membranes and tracers, we have a number of interesting phenomena. Substances can pass via the outer layer either through altered junctions because of inflammation or via micropinocytotic vesicles. On the other hand, observations on the inner layer reveal that this layer allows passage of substances to and from the inner ear giving the membrane interesting new roles of depurating and regulating inner ear fluids.

I believe that these aspects of otitis media are most interesting, and I firmly believe that systematic research in this area will help towards a better understanding of inner ear disease secondary to otitis media and, perhaps, may change some concepts in otology.

References

1. Paparella, M.M., Brady, D.R., and Hoel, R. Sensorineural hearing loss in chronic otitis media and mastoiditis. Trans Am Acad Ophtalmol Otolaryngol 74: 108–115, 1970.
2. Paparella, M.M., Goycoolea, M.V., Meyerhoff, W.L., and Shea, D. Endolymphatic hydrops and otitis media. Laryngoscope 89: 43–54, 1979.
3. Goycoolea, M.V. Pathogenesis of otitis media: An experimental study in the cat. Dissert Abstr Int 39: 132–210, 1978.
4. Goycoolea, M.V., Paparella, M.M., Juhn, S.K., and Carpenter, A.M. Pathogenesis of otitis media. A longitudinal study of cellular changes in otitis media. Otolaryngology 87: 685–700, 1979.
5. Goycoolea, M.V., Paparella, M.M., Juhn, S.K., and Carpenter, A.M. The cells involved in the middle ear defense system. Ann Otol Rhinol Laryngol (Suppl 68) 89: 121–128, 1980.
6. Goycoolea, M.V., Paparella, M.M., Juhn, S.K., and Carpenter, A.M. Oval and round window changes in otitis media: An experimental study in the cat. Surg Forum 29: 578–580, 1978.
7. Goycoolea, M.V., Paparella, M.M., Juhn, S.K., and Carpenter, A.M. Oval and round window changes in otitis media: Potential pathways from middle to inner ear. Laryngoscope 90: 1387–1391, 1980.
8. Carpenter, A.M., and Goycoolea, M.V. Morphometry of round window changes after Eustachian tube obstruction. Read before the Meeting of the Association for Research in Otolaryngology, St Petersburg, Fl., Jan. 23, 1979.
9. Goycoolea, M.V., Paparella, M.M., Goldberg, B., and Carpenter, A.M. Permeability of the round window membrane in otitis media. Arch Otol 106: 430–433, 1980.
10. Goycoolea, M.V., Paparella, M.M., Goldberg, B., Schlievert, P.M., and Carpenter, A.M. Permeability of the middle ear to staphylococcal pyrogenic exotoxin in otitis media. Internat J Pediatr Otolaryngol 1: 301–308, 1980.
11. Goldberg, B., Goycoolea, M.V., Schlievert, P.M., Shea, D., Schachern, P., Paparella, M.M., and Carpenter, A.M. Passage of albumin from middle to inner ear in otitis media in the chinchilla. Am J. Otol 2: 210–214, 1981.
12. Carpenter, A.M., Muchow, D., and Goycoolea, M.V. An ultrastructural study of the round window membrane. (Submitted for publication).

CHAPTER 2

Efficacy of Various Methods of Therapy for Otitis Media[1]

Charles D. Bluestone, M.D.[2]

Otitis media is the most frequent diagnosis made by physicians who care for children and is probably the most common condition in adults who are treated by otolaryngologists. (1). Acute otitis media is usually suppurative or purulent, but serous middle ear effusions may also have an acute onset. Chronic otitis media with effusion has many synonyms, including such terms as secretory, serous, nonsuppurative, and "glue ear." A chronic effusion may be serous, mucoid, or even purulent. In some instances, the eardrum may be retracted or collapsed without a middle ear effusion, which is termed *atelectasis* of the tympanic membrane, and is the result of persistent or intermittent negative middle ear pressure. It is often difficult to determine from the history and visual inspection of the tympanic membrane the precise type of otitis media present since in most patients, especially infants and young children, the disease is a continuum of the different stages. Some patients may have recurrent acute attacks without an apparent effusion in-between, whereas others may have only chronic otitis media with effusion, and still others may have recurrent acute episodes superimposed on a persistent middle ear effusion. Atelectasis of the tympanic membrane may represent the only pathology in some patients but in others, the condition can be present between episodes of otitis media with effusion. Chronic otitis media with perforation and otorrhea is one of the sequelae of acute or chronic otitis media with effusion.

EPIDEMIOLOGY

Infants and young children are at highest risk for the acquisition of otitis media, with the peak prevalence rate occurring between 6 and 36 months, and a lesser peak between 4 and 7 years (see Fig. 2.1) (2).

Figure 2.2 shows the findings in 2,565 children followed for the first 3 years of life. In this study, it was found that only 29% of infants failed to develop at least one attack of otitis media, whereas about one-third had three or more episodes (3). In addition, the study showed that after the first episode, 40% of children had a middle ear effusion that persisted for 4 weeks and 10% had an effusion which was still present at 3 months. Infants who develop otitis media with effusion in the first years of life have an increased risk of recurrent acute or chronic middle ear effusions.

The overall prevalence of the disease in children has been estimated at between 15–20% (4). However, the incidence and prevalence of the disease tend to decrease as a function of age after the age of 6 years. The incidence is higher in males, lower socioeconomic groups, Alaskan natives (Eskimos), American Indians, children with cleft palate and other craniofacial anomalies, and higher in whites than in blacks. The incidence is also higher in winter and early spring (5).

ACUTE OTITIS MEDIA WITH EFFUSION

In the classic description of this condition, a child who has an upper respiratory

---

[1] This study was supported, in part, by a grant from the National Institute of Neurological and Communicative Disorders and Stroke, 1P01-NS-16337.
[2] The author would like to thank Ms. Sandra Arjona for her assistance in the preparation of this manuscript.

4 Clinical Otology

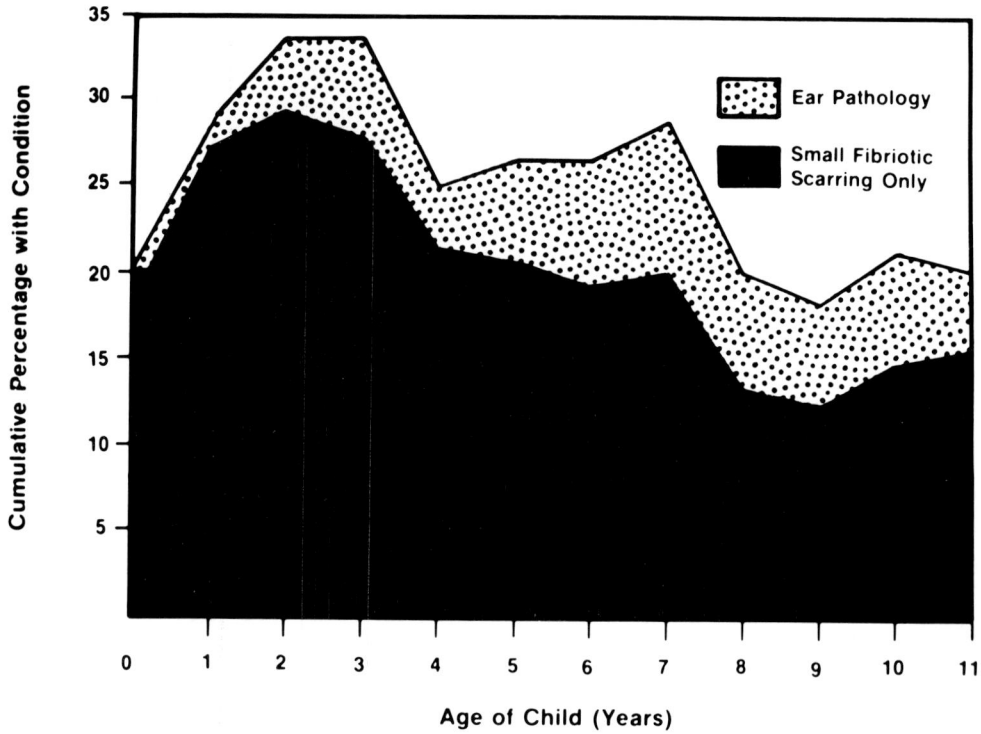

Figure 2.1. Point prevalence study of 2,158 infants and children in the Washington, D.C. area (2).

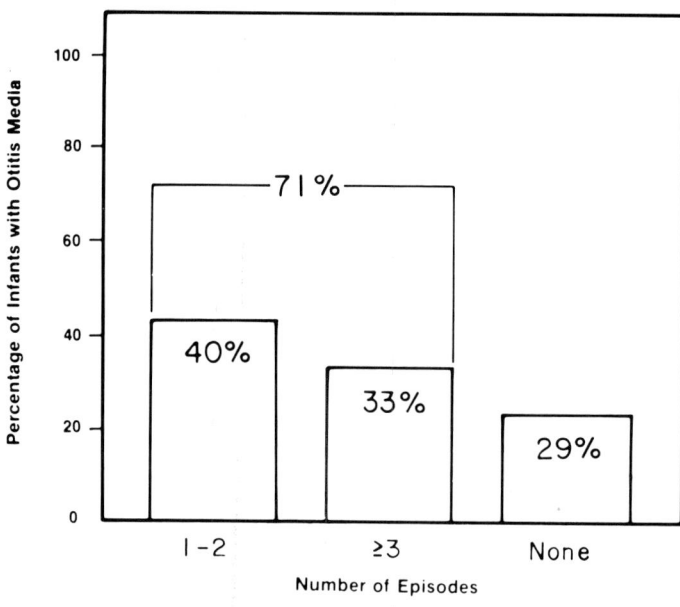

Figure 2.2. Study of epidemiology of otitis media from the Greater Boston Collaborative Media Program. Adapted from Teele et al. (3).

infection for several days suddenly develops otalgia, fever, and hearing loss. Examination with the pneumatic otoscope reveals a hyperemic, opaque, bulging tympanic membrane that has poor mobility. Purulent otorrhea may be present. However, earache and fever are not invariable concomitants of infection. Because of the variability of symptoms, an otoscopic examination should always be included in the evaluation of infants and children; those who have diminished or absent mobility and opacification of the tympanic membrane should be suspected of having a bacterial otitis media with effusion. Middle ear infection must be ruled out in any child with a "fever of undetermined origin." When the diagnosis of acute otitis media with effusion is in doubt, or when determination of the causative agent is desirable, aspiration of the middle ear should be performed.

Rational therapy for acute otitis media with effusion depends upon knowledge of the bacterial cause of the disease. The bacteria that have been cultured from middle ear effusions in children with acute otitis media have been shown to be the same found in the nasopharynx (6). *Streptococcus pneumoniae* has been cultured from approximately 30-40% of the effusions and is the most common causative agent in all age groups. *Haemophilus influenzae* causes about 20% of cases (Fig. 2.3). This proportion declines with increasing age but *H. influenzae* is still significant in *all* age groups. Recently, there has been an increasing percentage of *H. influenzae* strains, 15-30% that have been β-lactamase producing and therefore, ampicillin-resistant (7, 8). *Branhamella catarrhalis* is present in about 5%. Group A β-hemolytic streptococcus and *Staphylococcus aureus* account for 7 and 2% respectively. In about 25% of effusions, no bacteria are cultured. In neonates, approximately 20% of effusions may contain gram-negative enteric bacilli.

In patients with the classic signs and symptoms of acute otitis media antimicrobial therapy is the treatment of choice (Table 2.1) (9). Since the clinician rarely is certain of the causative organism before starting therapy for otitis media, ampicillin is the single most useful drug, and will usually be effective against the most commonly encountered bacteria. Oral ampicillin, 50-100 mg/kg/24 hrs, in four divided doses for 10-14 days is recommended. Amoxicillin, 20-40 mg/kg/24 hr, is probably equally effective and can be given in three divided doses. If the patient is allergic to the penicillins, then a combination of oral erythromycin, 50 mg/kg/24 hr, and triple sulfonamides, 100 mg/kg/24 hr (or sulfisoxazole, 150 mg/kg/24 hr), in four divided doses, is a suitable alternative. The combination of trimethoprim and sulfamethoxazole, 8-40 mg/kg/24 hr in two divided doses, also can initially be given to penicillin-sensitive individuals, but its effectiveness in the treatment of acute otitis media due to *Streptococcus pyogenes* is uncertain. A new cephalosporin, cefaclor, 40 mg/kg/24 hr, in three divided doses, appears to be a promising new antimicrobial agent for otitis media since it is effective against the common pathogens causing acute otitis media. The clinical efficacy of these antimicrobial agents is summarized in Table 2.2.

Additional supportive therapy, includ-

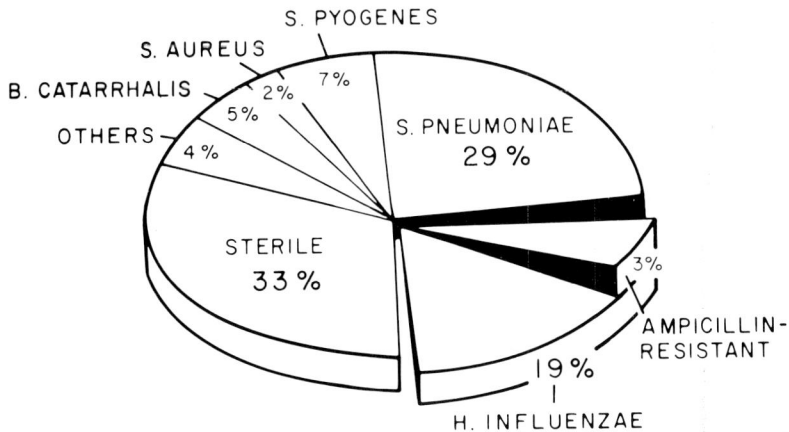

Figure 2.3. Bacteriology of acute otitis media. Middle ear aspirates were obtained by tympanocentesis from 83 ears of children 1-12 years of age (7).

ing analgesics, antipyretics, and local heat, will usually be helpful. In some instances, meperidine hydrochloride may also be required for sedation. The efficacy of antihistamines and decongestants in the treatment of acute otitis media has not been proven.

If the patient continues to have appreciable pain or persistent fever, or both, after 24-48 hr, tympanocentesis/myringotomy should be performed as a diagnostic and therapeutic procedure. At this stage, the presence of an effusion alone does not constitute a clinical failure. In patients with unusually severe earache, myringotomy may be performed initially in order to provide immediate relief.

When an unusual organism is cultured from a middle ear aspirate, sensitivity testing will help in the choice of antimicrobial agents. An example of this situation is an acute otitis media due to H. influenzae that is resistant to ampicillin. When this occurs or when the patient fails to improve clinically after the initial treatment with ampicillin or amoxicillin and a tympanocentesis/myringotomy is not performed, the initial antimicrobial should be changed since an ampicillin-resistant H. influenzae should be suspected. Erythromycin in combination with a sulfonamide, or trimethoprim-sulfamethoxazole, or cefaclor are appropriate choices at present.

All patients should be re-evaluated approximately 2 weeks after the institution of treatment. At this time, some patients will have had complete resolution of the middle ear effusion but in others complete clearing of the effusion may take 6 weeks or longer. Within 2-3 months, the tympanic membrane should be entirely nor-

Table 2.1
Therapeutic Results in Acute Otitis Media (9)

Drug	% Therapeutic Success	
	H. influenzae*	S. pneumoniae
Ampicillin	99	99
Penicillin V and Triple Sulfonamides	92	100
Erythromycin and Triple Sulfonamides	93	95
Penicillin V	42	100
Erythromycin	49	96
Triple Sulfonamides	83	76
Placebo	43	20

* Ampicillin sensitive

Table 2.2
Efficacy of Selected Antimicrobial Agents for the Common Pathogens in Acute Otitis Media*

Antimicrobial Agent	S. pneumoniae 35%	H. influenzae 20%		B. catarrhalis 5-10%	S. pyogenes 5-10%	S. aureus 2-10%
		Non β-lactamase 17%	β-lactamase 3%			
Ampicillin or Amoxicillin	+	+	−	±	+	±
Erythromycin-Sulfisoxazole	+	+	+	+	+	+
Trimethoprim-Sulfamethoxazole	+	+	+	±	−	±
Cefaclor	+	+	+	+	+	+

* Based on available data from clinical trials.
+ Effective.
± Effective for some strains but not all.
− Not effective.

mal. If complete resolution has occurred and the episode represents the only known attack, the patient may be discharged. However, periodic follow-up is indicated for patients who have had recurrent episodes.

RECURRENT ACUTE OTITIS MEDIA

It is not uncommon for children, especially infants, to have recurrent bouts of acute otitis media. Some children develop an acute episode with almost every respiratory tract infection, have more or less dramatic symptoms, respond well to therapy, and improve with advancing age. Others are more difficult, in that they have persistent middle ear effusion and suffer recurrent episodes of acute otitis media with effusion superimposed on the chronic disorder. The child with recurrent acute otitis media with effusion who completely clears between episodes may be managed as previously outlined. However, if the bouts are frequent and close together, further treatment, similar to that described for patients with chronic otitis media with effusion, is indicated. In many of these children, the underlying cause is not evident but myringotomy with insertion of middle ear tympanostomy tubes is frequently helpful. Prophylactic antimicrobials (a daily dose of ampicillin or sulfonamides) have been advocated as an alternative to tympanostomy tubes in children with recurrent acute otitis media with effusion who are free of effusion between attacks (Table 2.3). The efficacy of myringotomy with tympanostomy tube insertion and of chemoprophylaxis is as poorly established as is the usefulness of other forms of prevention, such as hyposensitization and adenoidectomy (10).

CHRONIC OTITIS MEDIA WITH EFFUSION

Chronic middle ear effusions may be thin (serous), thick (mucoid), or purulent in character. Pneumatic otoscopy will frequently reveal either a retracted or convex tympanic membrane. The membrane is usually opaque but when it is translucent, an air-fluid level or air bubbles may be seen and an amber or sometimes bluish fluid may be apparent in the middle ear. The mobility of the ear drum is almost always impaired. Occasionally, even when the middle ear is free of effusion, the tympanic membrane will be retracted and its mobility impaired. This finding usually indicates the presence of negative middle ear air pressure, which, when extreme, is termed "atelectasis of the tympanic membrane"; it may be accompanied by the same symptoms usually associated with otitis media with effusion. In both conditions, auditory acuity is usually decreased, and although systemic symptoms are usually absent, there may be behavioral disturbances owing to the child's inability to communicate adequately. A feeling of fullness in the ear, tinnitus, and even vertigo may be present. Audiometry may be helpful in establishing the diagnosis but is not a reliable indicator, because some patients, even with thick middle ear effusions, have fairly good hearing. Tympanometry is a more reliable diagnostic tool (11). A patient with chronic otitis media with effusion who has not received prior antimicrobial

Table 2.3
Chemoprophylaxis for Recurrent Acute Otitis Media with Effusion

Study	Drug	Duration	% Reduction
Ensign et al. (26) (Eskimos)	Sulfamethoxy-pyridazine	9 months	56 (Otorrhea)
Maynard et al. (27) (Eskimos)	Ampicillin	1 year	47 (Otorrhea)
Perrin et al. (28)	Sulfisoxazole	6 months	81
Biedel (29)	Sulfisoxazole	2 months (with URI)	71

therapy should be treated initially as a case of acute otitis media with effusion, since bacteria are frequently present (12, 13).

A study was conducted of 274 children who had recurrent acute or chronic otitis media with effusion (14). Figure 2.4 shows that 45% of the ears with effusion were found to contain bacteria and 11 percent bacteria that were "probable pathogens" (*S. pneumoniae, H. influenzae,* and *S. pyogenes*). Bacteria were also found in 40% of the ears without effusions. The type of organism found did not vary with the age of the patient studied or the season of the year. Pathogens have also been aspirated from young infants with chronic effusions (Fig. 2.5) (15). The significance of these bacteria in the etiology of recurrent acute or chronic otitis media with effusion remains to be demonstrated. However, the efficacy of antimicrobials, as well as decongestants and antihistamines, for chronic otitis media with effusion has not been proven. Occasionally, attempts at middle ear inflation by Valsalva's or Politzer's method are successful.

If the effusion persists for 8 weeks or longer, or if there have been frequent recurrences of episodes of acute otitis media with effusion, the patient requires further evaluation. Several avenues of investigation are open: a search for respiratory allergy may prove fruitful; a lateral roentgenogram of the nasopharynx may reveal adenoid tissue obstructing the nose and nasopharynx; immunological studies may be of value if other organs are involved (the lung, for example). In addition, more thorough physical examination may reveal abnormalities, such as submucous cleft palate or a tumor of the nasopharynx, that require definitive management.

For those patients in whom medical management has failed, myringotomy with aspiration of the middle ear fluid is indicated. Frequently, insertion of a tympanostomy tube may be necessary to allow the middle ear mucous membrane to return to normal and to prevent subsequent accumulation of effusion. Myringotomy and insertion of ventilation tubes may also be helpful in patients with atelectasis of the middle ear when significant symptoms—pain, hearing loss, vertigo, or tinnitus—are present. Ventilation tubes should be used to prevent permanent structural damage and cholesteatoma if a deep retraction pocket develops in the posterosuperior quadrant or in the attic (pars flaccida) portion of the tympanic membrane. Occasionally, troublesome otorrhea develops after the insertion of tympanostomy tubes. This can usually be treated successfully with ear drops containing neomycin, polymyxin, or colistin with hydrocortisone. Since these medications may be ototoxic, some physicians advocate the use of systemic antibiotics without the aural drops. In most children, otitis media with effusion is usually self-limiting and will improve with advancing age, but in se-

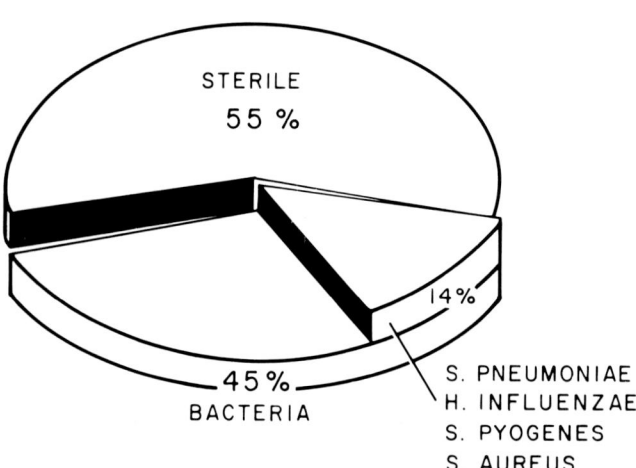

Figure 2.4. Bacteriology of ears of children 1–16 years of age who had chronic or recurrent otitis media with effusion (14).

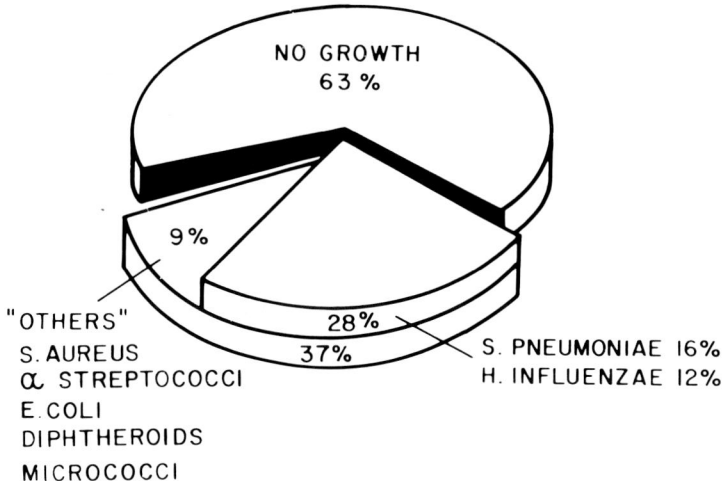

Figure 2.5. Bacteriology of chronic or recurrent otitis media with effusion in 50 infants (100 ears) 1–12 months of age (15).

lected cases, allergic hyposensitization and adenoidectomy may be beneficial; however, the efficacy of these methods of management has not been established. Tonsillectomy (in the absence of documented recurrent tonsillitis) does not seem to alter the course of otitis of any type and probably should not be performed in conjunction with adenoidectomy for these conditions (16).

Since otitis media with effusion is universal in the infant with an unrepaired cleft palate and very common after surgical repair of the palate, tympanostomy tubes should be inserted when a chronic effusion is present to prevent the complications and sequelae of otitis media (17).

Atelectasis of the Tympanic Membrane-Middle Ear and High Negative Middle Ear Pressure

Atelectasis of the tympanic membrane can be either acute or chronic, generalized or localized, mild or severe, and may or may not be associated with abnormal negative middle ear pressure. Retraction of the tympanic membrane may be secondary to the presence of high negative pressure. However, a flaccid, atelectatic tympanic membrane may not be associated with high negative intratympanic pressure: the abnormal negative pressure may have been the original cause of such a condition of the membrane but may no longer be present. Localized atelectasis or a retraction pocket may be seen in the area of a healed perforation or at the site where a tympanostomy tube had been inserted. A retraction pocket in the posterosuperior portion of the pars tensa or a pars flaccida retraction pocket is more frequently associated with the development of more serious sequelae (ossicular necrosis or cholesteatoma) than is a retraction pocket in other areas of the tympanic membrane (see Fig. 2.6) (18). These variations should be kept in mind when deciding how to manage atelectasis.

If a chronic middle ear effusion is present concurrently with atelectasis, then the child should be treated as previously outlined for patients with chronic otitis media with effusion. However, whether or not a middle ear effusion is present, if a chronic severe retraction pocket of the posterosuperior area of the pars tensa or of the pars flaccida or both is present, a myringotomy and insertion of a tympanostomy tube should be performed to prevent possible irreversible changes in the middle ear. After insertion of a tympanostomy tube, the tympanic membrane in the area of the retraction pocket should return to a more neutral position within several weeks or months, but if the retraction area remains

10 Clinical Otology

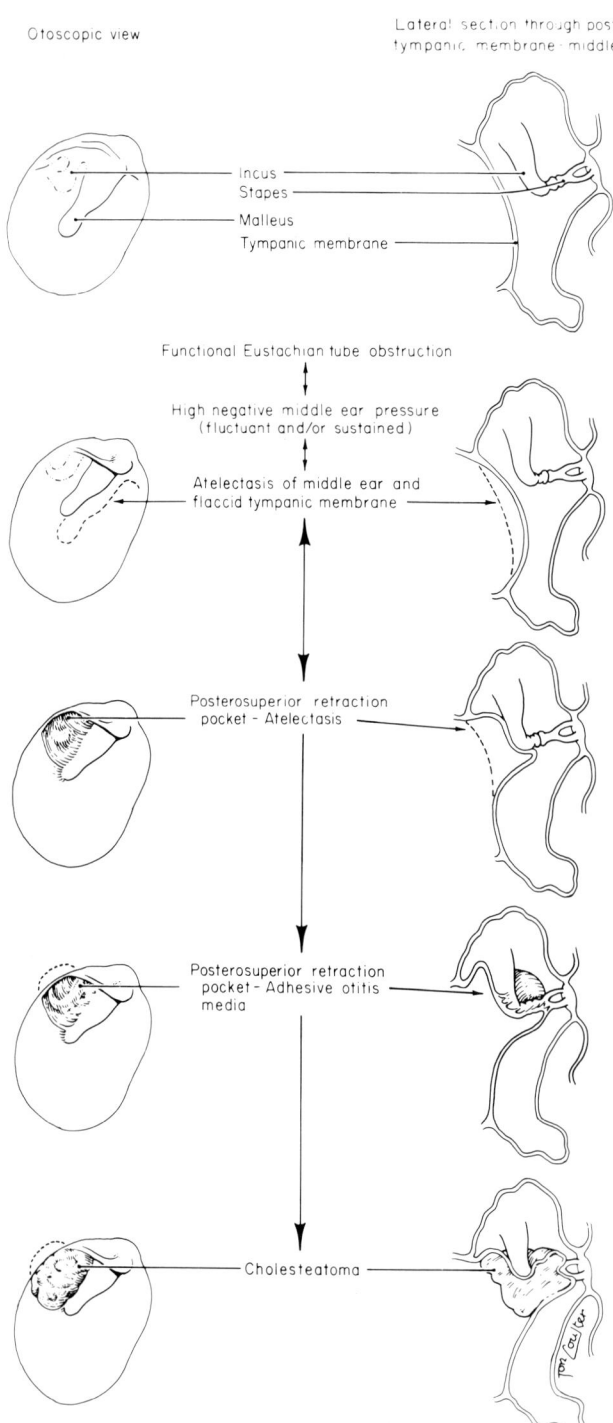

Figure 2.6. Sequence of events in the pathogenesis of a cholesteatoma in the posterosuperior portion of the pars tensa.

adherent to the ossicles or middle ear or both, then adhesive otitis media is present, and a tympanoplasty should be considered to prevent further progression of the disease process (such as ossicular necrosis or cholesteatoma formation, or both). Even though this method of management has not been tested in appropriately controlled clinical trials and the natural history of retraction pockets in these areas has not been studied adequately, this method of management would appear to be reasonable at present.

For less severe cases in which the atelectasis of the tympanic membrane is apparently not associated with a middle ear effusion and a retraction pocket is not present in the posterosuperior portion or pars flaccida, the management options become less obvious and more controversial. Generalized atelectasis, or even a localized area which is retracted for only a short time (acute retraction) is usually secondary to transient high negative middle ear pressure associated with an acute upper respiratory tract infection (and occasionally due to barotrauma). This condition is quite common in children and usually is self-limited. No specific treatment should be directed toward the middle ear unless the patient complains of severe otalgia, hearing loss, tinnitis, or vertigo. The atelectasis (and high negative intratympanic pressure) and associated symptoms, if present, will usually subside when the acute upper respiratory tract infection disappears. Treatment at this time should be directed toward relief of the nasal symptoms. Topical or systemic nasal decongestants may provide relief of these symptoms and may also decongest the Eustachian tube, although their effectiveness in this latter area has not yet been shown. If the symptoms become severe enough, a myringotomy may be necessary to provide relief by returning middle ear pressure to ambient. Inflation of the Eustachian tube-middle ear employing the methods of Valsalva or Politzer (see Figs. 2.7 and 2.8), or

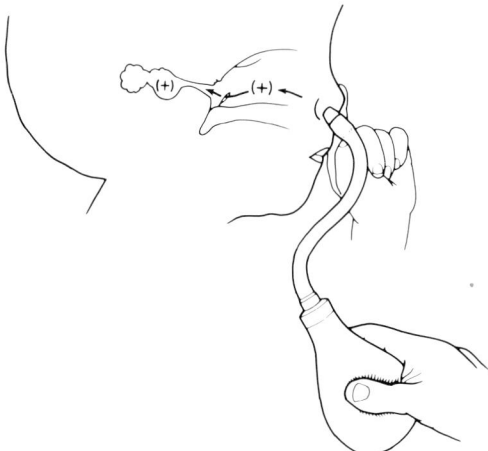

Figure 2.8. Politzer method of inflation of Eustachian tube-middle ear.

Eustachian tube catheterization has been advocated and has merit from a physiological standpoint. However, unwanted bacteria from the nasopharynx could be insufflated into the middle ear during the procedure, which could result in an acute otitis media.

When the atelectasis is chronic and there is no evidence of a deep retraction pocket in the posterosuperior quadrant or pars flaccida, a thorough search should be made for underlying etiology as described previously for recurrent acute or chronic otitis media with effusion. If none is found, then the management options include only watchful waiting and active treatment. The decision for or against treatment should rest on the presence or absence of other, associated symptoms, and whether or not there is abnormal negative pressure within the middle ear. The presence of persistent or transient otalgia, hearing loss, vertigo, or tinnitus which is troublesome to the patient warrants active treatment. For chronic atelectasis, in this case, a trial with a topical or systemic nasal decongestant with or without an antihistamine may be helpful; however, this type of treatment is often disappointing. Inflation of the Eustachian tube-middle ear may provide temporary relief but usually must be repeated for permanent control of the symptoms and to maintain the tympanic membrane in a more normal position. For most children, a myringotomy with insertion of a

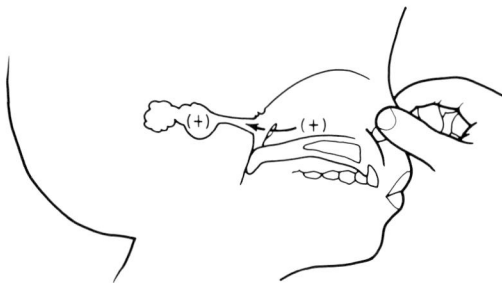

Figure 2.7. Valsalva method of inflation of Eustachian tube-middle ear.

tympanostomy tube will usually be necessary to provide long-term relief. The procedure will prevent the sustained or transient high negative pressure secondary to Eustachian tube dysfunction which is responsible for the active retraction of the tympanic membrane. If the severely atelectatic tympanic membrane does not return to a more normal position after the insertion of the tympanostomy tube, or the tube cannot be inserted due to lack of a suitable aerated space within the middle ear, a tympanoplasty should be considered.

When a flaccid tympanic membrane is passively collapsed upon the ossicles and middle ear and high negative middle ear pressure is not present, the nonsurgical and surgical management options described previously may not be effective in restoring the tympanic membrane to a more normal position. Fortunately, symptoms of high negative middle ear pressure and Eustachian tube dysfunction are frequently absent so that no treatment may be necessary. Even myringotomy and tympanostomy tube insertion may not be beneficial since the tympanic membrane is no longer actively being retracted by high negative middle ear pressure. In addition, at this stage, adhesive otitis media may also be present so that portions of the tympanic membrane may be adherent to the middle ear. In such cases, there are two management options: tympanoplasty or periodic (once or twice a year) observation.

Eustachian Tube Dysfunction

Otitis media with effusion and atelectasis with or without effusion are usually the result of dysfunction of the Eustachian tube. However, abnormal function of the Eustachian tube may cause otological symptoms without an apparent effusion or severe atelectasis. The tympanic membrane may have a normal appearance and mobility may be unimpaired when tested with a pneumatic otoscope or by tympanometry. Two types of Eustachian tube dysfunction can be present: obstruction or abnormal patency. When the Eustachian tube is obstructed but no effusion is present, the tube periodically opens to ventilate the middle ear cavity but at less frequent intervals than normal; in this case, high negative intratympanic pressure may be present for relatively long, but transient periods. This type of intermittent middle ear ventilation may cause periods of otalgia, a feeling of fullness or pressure, hearing loss, popping and snapping noises, tinnitus, and even vertigo. Management of this situation should be similar to that described for generalized atelectasis of the tympanic membrane. If the condition is present only during an acute upper respiratory tract infection, medical treatment should be directed toward relief of the nasal congestion. If the symptoms are of a chronic nature, a search for an underlying cause should be attempted, and if found, appropriate management instituted. If no underlying cause is uncovered, then a trial with a decongestant or antihistamine, or both, may be helpful, or Eustachian tube-middle ear inflation may be tried, but if the nonsurgical methods are not successful, then myringotomy and insertion of a tympanostomy tube may be necessary.

At the other end of the spectrum of Eustachian tube dysfunction is abnormal patency. In its extreme form, the hyperpatent Eustachan tube is open even at rest, i.e., patulous. Lesser degrees of abnormal patency result in a semipatulous Eustachian tube that is closed at rest but has low tubal resistance to airflow in comparison to the normal tube. A patulous Eustachian tube may be due to abnormal tube geometry or to a decrease in extramural pressure, such as occurs as a result of weight loss or possibly as a result of mural or intraluminal changes. These latter may be seen when the extracellular fluid is altered by medical treatment of another, unrelated condition. Interruption of the innervation of the tensor veli palatini muscle has also been shown to be a cause of a hyperpatent Eustachian tube.

Clinically, a patulous Eustachian tube may be present in adolescents and adults but is rarely seen in young children. The patient frequently complains of hearing his/her own breathing in the ear or of autophony. Otoscopic examination reveals a tympanic membrane that moves medially on inspiration and laterally on expiration; the movement can be exaggerated with forced respiration. The condition is relieved when the patient is recumbent, since Eustachian tube extramural pressure is increased by paratubal venous engorgement in this position. The patient should therefore be examined in the sitting position. The diagnosis can also be made by measuring the impedance of the middle ear (19). A tympanogram should be obtained while the patient is breathing normally, and a second one obtained while the patient holds his breath. Fluctuation in the tympanometric line should coincide with breathing. The fluctuation can be exaggerated by asking the patient to occlude one nostril and close the mouth during forced inspiration and expiration, or by performing the Toynbee or Valsalva maneuver.

Management of a patulous Eustachian tube depends on first determining the etiology of the problem. If the symptoms are of relatively short duration, the condition may subside without any active treatment. In children and teenagers, this condition is usually self-limited and probably related to changes in the structure and function of the Eustachian tube and adjacent areas secondary to rapid growth and development. When a medication can be identified as the agent responsible, cessation of the medication usually alleviates the problem. However, in most instances, the condition is idiopathic. When the symptoms are disturbing and the condition is chronic, active treatment is indicated. A myringotomy with insertion of a tympanostomy tube may be performed but usually does not alter the symptoms in most cases and occasionally will result in increasing the patient's discomfort. Insufflation of powders into the Eustachian tube (Bezold's treatment—insufflation of boric and salicylic acid powder), and instillation of 2% iodine or 5% trichloracetic acid solution have also been advocated. Infusion of an absorbable gelatin sponge solution has also been suggested, as has injection of polytetrafluoroethylene (Teflon^R) into the paratubal area, but all of these methods have major disadvantages. They are, for the most part, irreversible and may not improve the condition or may provide only temporary relief. Total obstruction of the Eustachian tube can also be a complication.

At present, the most logical choice for relief when the discomfort becomes severe is a procedure that would alleviate the symptoms simply reversibly and without untoward reactions. The technique described below has been found to fulfill these criteria and has been successful in relieving the symptoms of patulous Eustachian tube (20). An anterior tympanotomy approach was used to insert an indwelling intravenous catheter with flared tip (Medicut^R) into the protympanic, or bony, portion of the Eustachian tube (see Fig. 2.9). The flared end of the catheter rests in the middle ear end of the Eustachian tube. Prior to insertion, the lumen of the catheter had been filled with methyl methacrylate

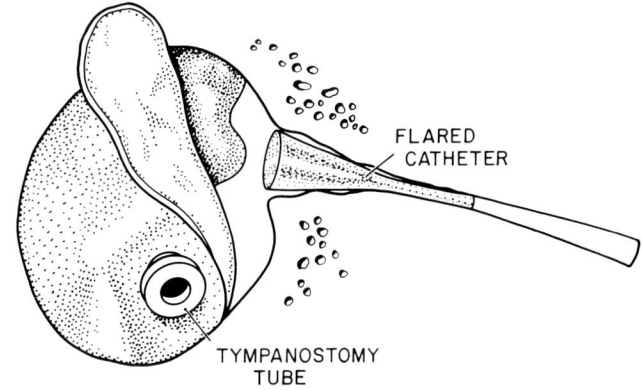

Figure 2.9. Illustration of technique of placement of indwelling catheter used to obstruct a patulous Eustachian tube.

to prevent the passage of air through the catheter; thus, the catheter occludes the Eustachian tube. Following insertion of the catheter, a tympanostomy tube is inserted into the tympanic membrane to aerate the middle ear through the membrane. Even though spontaneous extrusion of the tympanostomy tube occurred in 2 subjects, their middle ears have remained aerated with relief of symptoms and without development of high negative pressure or effusion or both. The catheter most likely did not totally obstruct the Eustachian tube, and adequate ventilation of the middle ear was provided around the catheter. Only a small number of patients have had the procedure but the results have been gratifying. The longest follow-up has been 3 years.

The indwelling Eustachian tube catheter can be removed at any time, especially if and when the etiology of this most perplexing otologic problem is uncovered and a nonsurgical or surgical method of management is shown to be more efficacious. In the meantime, this method of Eustachian tube obstruction has been shown to be effective in providing relief of symptoms of a patulous Eustachian tube.

COMPLICATIONS AND SEQUELAE OF OTITIS MEDIA

Today, the intracranial suppurative complications of otitis media with effusion are relatively uncommon except in neglected cases. However, the complications and sequelae that occur within the aural cavity and adjacent structures of the temporal bone are more common and awareness of their possible existence is essential in management of children with otitis media with effusion. Even though many of these less serious conditions may not threaten life (as when there is an intracranial extension of the disease), the quality of life may be severely affected, making prevention imperative.

Hearing loss is by far the most prevalent complication and morbid outcome of otitis media with effusion, and may be caused by one or more of the intra-aural complications or sequelae. To a varying degree, fluctuating or persistent loss of hearing is always associated with acute or chronic otitis media with effusion. The presence of high negative pressure within the middle ear (atelectasis), in the absence of an effusion, can also be associated with a significant hearing loss. The audiogram usually reveals a mild to moderate conductive loss. However, there may be a sensorineural component, generally attributed to the effect of increased tension and stiffness of the round window membrane. This hearing loss is usually reversible with resolution of the effusion, but permanent conductive hearing loss can result from irreversible changes secondary to recurrent acute or chronic inflammation, e.g., adhesive otitis, tympanosclerosis, or ossicular discontinuity. Irreparable sensorineural loss may also occur, presumably as the result of spread of infection through the round or oval window membrane (21). Audiometry can be reliably performed in children over 3 years of age, but children under 3 years are the group at highest risk for effusions and associated hearing loss and in these patients, standard audiometric assessment is difficult to perform reliably. Whenever an otitis media with effusion is diagnosed clinically or by tympanometry, there is a concurrent hearing loss (22). The relation between persistent or episodic hearing loss and impairment in the cognitive, language, or emotional development of children has been reported (23–25). However, the degree and duration of the hearing loss required to produce such deficits have not been defined.

SUMMARY

1. Otitis media with effusion and its complications and sequelae are one of the most common disorders encountered by the otolaryngologist.
2. Pathogenesis related to Eustachian tube dysfunction.
3. Etiology primarily bacterial (*S. pneumoniae* 40%, *H. influenzae* 20%). Bacteria also present in chronic otitis media with effusion ("secretory otitis").
4. *H. influenzae* present in all age groups, and 15–30% are ampicillin-resistant.
5. Diagnosis by pneumatic otoscopy or tympanometry, or both.

6. Tympanocentesis and myringotomy important diagnostic—therapeutic procedures in selected patients.

7. Ampicillin (or amoxicillin) initial therapy of choice.

8. Erythromycin and sulfonamide, trimethoprim-sulfamethoxazole or cefaclor recommended for those who have poor clinical response to initial antimicrobial therapy.

9. Efficacy yet to be shown for antimicrobial prophylaxis, decongestants, antihistamines, and adenoidectomy with or without tonsillectomy, however, tympanostomy tubes can be helpful in restoring hearing to within normal limits.

10. Atelectasis of the tympanic membrane, especially when localized to the posterosuperior quadrant of the pars tensa or pars flaccida may lead to the development of cholesteatoma, making prevention imperative. Tympanotomy tube insertion can successfully return the tympanic membrane to the normal position in many cases.

11. Attendant conductive hearing loss may be related to abnormalities in cognition, language, and learning in children.

References

1. Koch, H., and Dennison, N.J. Office visits to pediatricians, National Ambulatory Medical Service, National Center for Health Statistics, Washington, D.C., 1974.
2. Kessner, D., Snow, C.K., and Singer, T. Assessment of medical care for children: Contrasts in health care status. Vol. 3, Washington, D.C., Institute of Medicine, National Academy of Sciences, 1974.
3. Teele, W.W., Klein, J.O., and Rosner, B.A. Epidemiology of otitis media in children. *Ann Otol Rhinol Laryngol 89 (Suppl 68):* 5–6, 1980.
4. Avery, A.D., Lelah, T., Solomon, N.E., Harris, J.L., Brook, R.H., Greenfield, S., Ware, J.E., and Avery, C.H. Quality of medical care assessment using outcome measures: Eight disease-specific applications. Prepared for the Health Resources Administration, Department of Health, Education and Welfare (R-2021/2-HEW) by the Rand Corporation, Santa Monica, California 90406, August, 1976.
5. Bluestone, CD. The Ear. In: *Nelson's Textbook of Pediatrics,* Vaughan, V.C., McKay, R.J., and Behrman, R.E. (Eds.), 11th ed., W.B. Saunders Co., Philadelphia, 1979.
6. Bluestone, C.D., and Shurin, P. Middle ear disease in children: Pathogenesis, diagnosis and management. *Pediatr Clin North Am 21:* 379–400, 1974.
7. Bluestone, C.D., Beery, Q.C., Michaels, R.M., Zanotti, M.L., Stool, S.E., Grundfast, K.M., Wright, C.M., and Mandel, E.M. Efficacy of cefaclor compared to amoxicillin in the treatment of acute otitis media with effusion in infants and children: A preliminary report. *Post Grad Med J 55 (Suppl 4):* 42–49, 1979.
8. Paradise, J.L. Otitis media in infants and children. *Pediatrics 65:* 917–943, 1980.
9. Howie, V.M., and Ploussard, J.H. The "in vivo sensitivity test"—Bacteriology of middle ear exudate. *Pediatrics 44:* 940, 1969.
10. Bluestone, C.D. Assessment of Eustachian tube function. In: *Handbook of Clinical Impedance Audiometry,* American Electromedics Corp., New York, 1975.
11. Bluestone, C.D., Beery, Q.C., and Paradise, J.L. Audiometry and tympanometry in relation to middle ear effusions in children. *Laryngoscope 83:* 594–604, 1973.
12. Healy, G.B., and Teele, D.W. The microbiology of chronic middle ear effusions in children. *Laryngoscope 87:* 1472–1478, 1977.
13. Liu, Y.S., Lim, D.S., and Lang, R.W. Chronic middle ear effusions: Immunological and bacteriological investigations. *Arch Otolaryngol 101:* 278–286, 1975.
14. Riding, K.H., Bluestone, C.D., Michaels, R.H., Cantekin, E.I., Doyle, W.J., and Poziviak, C.S. Microbiology of recurrent and chronic otitis media with effusion. *J Pediatr 93:* 739–743, 1978.
15. Stanievich, J.F., Bluestone, C.D., Lima, J.A., Michaels, R.H., Rohn, D., and Effron, M.Z. Microbiology of chronic and recurrent otitis media with effusion in young infants. *Int J Ped Otorhinolaryngol* (In Press) 1981.
16. McKee, W.J. The part played by adenoidectomy in the combined operation of tonsillectomy with adenoidectomy: Second part of a controlled study in children. *Br J Prev Soc Med 17:* 133–140, 1963.
17. Paradise, J.L., and Bluestone, C.D. Early treatment of infants with cleft palate. *Pediatrics 53:* 48–54, 1974.
18. Bluestone, C.D., Cantekin, E.I., Beery, Q.C., and Stool, S.E. Function of the Eustachian tube related to surgical management of acquired aural cholesteatoma in children. *Laryngoscope 87:* 1155–1163, 1978.
19. Bluestone, C.D. Assessment of Eustachian tube function. In: *Clinical Impedance Audiometry.* Jerger J., and Northern J. (Eds.), American Electromedics Corp., Acton, MA, 1980.
20. Bluestone, C.D., and Cantekin, E.I. Management of the patulous Eustachian tube. *Laryngoscope 91:* 149–152, 1981.
21. Paparella, M.M., Oda, M., Hiraida, F., and Brady, D. Pathology of sensorineural hearing loss in otitis media. *Ann Otol Rhinol Laryngol 81:* 632, 1972.
22. Olmstead, R.W. A study of the pattern of hearing in children following acute otitis media. *Am J Dis Child 100:* 772, 1960.
23. Fisher, B. The social and emotional adjustment of children with impaired hearing attending ordinary classes. *Pa J Ed Psychol 36:* 319–321, 1966.
24. Holm, V.A., and Kunze, L.H. Effect of chronic otitis media on language and speech development. *Pediatrics 48:* 833–839, 1969.

25. Lewis, N. Otitis media and linguistic competence. *Arch Otolaryngol 102:* 387–390, 1976.
26. Ensign, R.R., Urbanich, E.M., and Moran, J. Prophylaxis for otitia media in an Indian population. *Am J Publ Health 50:* 195–199, 1960.
27. Maynard, J.E., Fleshman, J.K., and Tschopp, C.F. Otitis media in Alaskan Eskimo children: Prospective evaluation of chemoprophylaxis. *JAMA 219:* 597–599, 1972.
28. Perrin, J.M., Charney, E., MacWhinney, J.B. Jr., et al. Sulfisoxazole chemoprophylaxis for recurrent otitis media: A double-blind crossover study in pediatric practice. *N Engl J Med 291:* 667, 1974.
29. Biedel, C.S. Modification of recurrent otitis media by short-term sulfonamide therapy. *Am J Dis Child 132:* 681, 1978.

CHAPTER 3

Tympanostomy Tube Therapy for Otitis Media[1]

William L. Meyerhoff, M.D., Ph.D.

Middle ear effusion (MEE) is the most common cause of hearing loss in children. The hearing loss imposed by this condition, although usually transient, appears to be significant enough to cause psychosocial and educational sequelae. In spite of its frequency and potential morbidity, the best treatment for MEE is yet to be agreed upon and some clinicians believe that no treatment at all is needed. The spectrum of proposed therapies for MEE include systemic and topical decongestants, antihistamines, autoinflation, allergic hyposensitization, antimicrobials, anti-inflammatory agents, and surgery. The surgery most frequently employed is myringotomy and tympanostomy tube insertion. The proponents of this form of therapy cite the immediate improvement in hearing as their main accomplishment and a decreased incidence of recurrent acute purulent otitis media as well as decreased incidence of middle ear and inner ear sequelae as additional potential benefits.

Those who oppose tympanostomy tube insertion do not deny the immediate hearing gain which accompanies this procedure but believe that the operation cannot be justified on the basis of potential intraoperative risks and long-term scarring of the tympanic membrane. The cost of tympanostomy tube insertion has never been adequately compared to the cost of nonsurgical treatment of the otitis prone patient and the value of preserved or restored hearing is incalculable. For this reason, cost alone cannot be a determining factor.

POTENTIAL DISADVANTAGES OF TYMPANOSTOMY TUBE THERAPY

Several reports have appeared in the literature describing intraoperative surgical complications that have occurred in the course of myringotomy and tympanostomy tube insertion. Although aberrant carotid artery in the middle ear cleft was reported as early as 1899 by Max (1), a report of injury to the internal carotid artery by myringotomy could not be found until 1971. Ten years later (1981), Goodman and Cohen (2) described an additional case in which an aberrant internal carotid artery was lacerated with a myringotomy knife. The child subsequently exsanguinated despite attempts at hemostasis. The author has experienced a similar situation in which the hemorrhage that followed myringotomy incision in the internal carotid artery was fortunately controlled and the child recovered without sequelae.

Additional, but less catastrophic operative complications that may occur during myringotomy and tympanostomy tube insertion include laceration of a high jugular bulb and dural laceration in the case of a dehiscent tegmen tympani. Page (3) was probably first to report laceration of a dehiscent jugular bulb during myringotomy. Graham (4) reported several cases in which a dehiscent jugular bulb was identified in the course of otologic surgery, three of which suffered jugular bulb injury. The jugular bulb is dehiscent in the hypotympanum in approximately 6% of all temporal bones making such an injury potentially a more frequent complication than has been identified in the past. Al-

---

[1]This chapter was presented at the Third International Symposium, Minneapolis, Minnesota, September, 1981.

though bleeding is profuse with such an injury, it is more easily controlled than that which emanates from the internal carotid artery and long-term sequelae are rare in experienced hands.

Dural laceration is another possible complication of myringotomy when there is almost total absence of the tegmen tympani and prolapsed contents of the middle cranial fossa into the middle ear cleft. Such a case was reported in which a tympanostomy tube was actually placed through the myringotomy incision in the dura and meningitis ensued. This author experienced a similar case in a 2-year-old child with Downs' syndrome but the situation was recognized upon myringotomy and antimicrobials were begun and the external auditory canal was dressed without sequelae. Conceivable intraoperative complications of myringotomy and tympanostomy tube insertion not yet reported in the literature include fatal or morbid complications of inhalation anesthesia, facial nerve paralysis, and ossicular fracture or dislocation.

The most frequent postoperative complication of tympanostomy tube insertion is otitis media with otorrhea. This complication may occur early (first 10 days) or late (after 10 days). The most frequent long-term sequelae of tympanostomy tube insertion are changes in the tympanic membrane.

Early postoperative otorrhea occurs in up to 10% of cases and is related to the underlying condition for which the procedure was performed and the nature of the MEE. This complication can be reduced in frequency, somewhat, by preoperative sterilization of the external auditory canal and proper selection of materials used in the tube design. Sterilization of the external auditory canal can be accomplished in over 90% of the cases by instilling 70% alcohol in the external auditory canal for a period of 90 seconds. As far as tube design is concerned, it has been shown experimentally that teflon appears to be more resistant to infection than silastic.

When early postoperative otorrhea does occur, it usually responds to optical therapy in combination with systemic antimicrobials. On rare occasion, tympanostomy tube removal will be necessary. Late postoperative otorrhea may be the result of contamination by water in the external auditory canal or a manifestation of an isolated new episode of purulent otitis media. Again, topical therapy and systemic antimicrobials are usually sufficient treatment.

Long-term changes in the tympanic membrane following tympanostomy tube insertion have been identified in up to 60% of cases and include tympanosclerosis, atrophy, and occasionally persistent perforation. Little attempt has been made to separate these occurrences, however, from those that are part of the otitis process itself and, in most instances, no clinical significance has been attached to them. Cholesteatoma has been identified in about 0.5% of ears that previously have had tympanostomy tubes inserted but, this occurrence cannot necessarily be attributed to the tympanostomy tube itself as opposed to the otitis process.

POTENTIAL BENEFITS OF TYMPANOSTOMY TUBE INSERTION

The conductive hearing loss of MEE averages approximately 22–27 dB in the speech frequencies and is reversed, almost entirely, by tympanostomy tube insertion. A conductive hearing loss of this magnitude, even when intermittent and temporary, results in psychosocial and educational handicaps. Needleman (5) has identified linguistic problems and strained relationships between parents and children when the latter suffered the hearing loss of otitis media and these linguistic problems and strained relationships eventually resulted in detriment of the child's social development and academic success. It was similarly concluded by the Communicative Disorders Program of the National Institute for Neurological Disease and Stroke (1979) that the conductive hearing loss of recurrent and persistent MEE does, indeed, adversely affect speech, language, congnition, and socialization of the developing child.

In addition to their beneficial effect on the conductive hearing loss of MEE tympanostomy tube insertion appears to reduce the incidence of recurrent acute purulent otitis media in properly selected cases. Gebhardt (6) prospectively studied the effect of this treatment on the frequency of acute purulent otitis media in 95 children 36 months of age and under with refractory acute purulent otitis media. He randomly divided these children into two treatment protocols, one receiving prolonged, prophylactic antimicrobials and the other receiving tympanostomy tubes. The post-therapeutic incidence of recurrent acute purulent otitis media in the former group was significantly greater than that in the latter group. Further, it appears from animal experiments that the middle ear and inner ear morbidity that result from acute purulent otitis media are lessened by the presence of tympanostomy tubes.

CONCLUSIONS

The cost effectiveness of tympanostomy tubes as a treatment for otitis media is difficult to determine. Surgical and anesthetic fees have not been compared to nonsurgical outpatient care of the otitis prone patient and the value of hearing restoration and preservation is, at present, impossible to assess. Although the incidence and severity of anesthetic and surgical complications associated with tympanostomy tube insertion are not precisely known, they do not appear to be significant enough to warrant these potential problems as deterrant factors for this procedure. In spite of evidence that tympanic membrane changes occur following tympanostomy tube insertion, there is little evidence that separates those postoperative tympanic membrane changes from those that are secondary to the process of otitis media itself. The cause and effect of postoperative otorrhea and middle ear inflammation is not well understood. Whether this otorrhea is stimulated by the tympanostomy tube or whether the tympanostomy tube merely serves as an escape for effusion resulting from other local and regional factors is speculative. The incidence of postoperative otorrhea can be decreased if the external auditory canal is properly sterilized and the least reactive material is used. Whether tympanostomy tubes increase or decrease the incidence of inner ear disease in otitis media is not known.

There is no doubt that tympanostomy tubes usually correct the conductive hearing loss imposed by MEE and presumably, the educational and psychological ramifications. The incidence of recurrent acute otitis media appears clinically to be reduced by the insertion of tympanostomy tubes and the results of animal experiments suggest that tympanostomy tubes also reduce the incidence and severity of middle ear sequelae in otitis media.

For these reasons, it is concluded that, in the hands of capable surgeons and competent anesthetists and anesthesiologists, tympanostomy tube insertion as a treatment for otitis media is almost free of intraoperative and postoperative complications while eliminating the conductive hearing loss and reducing the incidence of recurrent acute otitis media and its sequelae. With proper patient selection (intractable MEE), appropriate treatment of associated conditions (maxillary sinusititis, allergy, nasopharyngeal infections), sterilization of the external auditory canal, and the use of least easily infected materials tympanostomy tube insertion is an efficacious procedure.

References

1. Max, E. Die bedeutung arteria carotitis interna in der hals. Nason Ohrenheilkinde. Msch Ohrenheilk, pp. 251, 1899.
2. Goodman, R.S., and Cohen, N.L. Aberrant internal carotid artery in the middle ear. Ann Otol 90: 67–69, 1981.
3. Page, J.R. A case of probable injury to the jugular bulb following myringotomy in an infant 10 months old. Ann Otol Rhinol Laryngol 23: 161, 1914.
4. Graham, M.D. The jugular bulb. Arch Otolaryngol 101: 560–564, 1975.
5. Needelman, H. Effects of hearing loss from early recurrent otitis media on speech and language development. In Hearing Loss in Children. Jaffe, B.F. (Eds), University Park Press, Baltimore, MD, 1977.
6. Gebhart, D. Tympanostomy tubes in the otitis media prone child. Presented at the 84th Annual

Meeting of the American Laryngology, Rhinology, and Otological Society, Vancouver, Canada, May 14, 1981.
7. Armstrong, B.W. A new treatment for chronic secretory otitis media. *Arch Otolaryngol 59:* 653, 1954.
8. Buckingham, R.A. Cholesteatoma and chronic otitis media following middle ear intubation. Presented at the Meeting of the Middle Section of the American Laryngological, Rhinological, and Otological Society, Inc., Oklahoma City, Oklahoma, January 23, 1981.
9. Goldman, N.C., Singleton, G.T., and Holly E.H. Aberrant internal carotid artery. *Arch Otolaryngol 94:* 269–273, 1971.
10. Hanson, D.G., and Ulvestad, R.F. Otitis media and child development. *Ann Otol Rhinol Laryngol* (Suppl. 60) *88:* 000, 1979.
11. Herzon, F. Tympanostomy tubes: Infectious complications. *Arch Otolaryngol 106:* 645–647, 1980.
12. McLelland, C.A. Incidence of complications from use of tympanostomy tubes. *Arch Otolaryngol 106:* 97–99, 1980.
13. Meyerhoff, W.L. Use of tympanostomy tubes in otitis media. Presented to the American Otological Society, Vancouver, May, 1981.
14. Meyerhoff W.L., and Giebink, G.S. Current concepts in otitis media. In *Family Practice Rev,* Academic Press, 1980.
15. Meyerhoff, W.L., Giebink, G.S., Shea, D.A., and Le, C.T. Effect of tympanostomy tubes on the pathogenesis of acute otitis media. *Am J Otolaryngol,* February, 1981.

CHAPTER 4

Status of Tonsillectomy and Adenoidectomy in the Treatment of Otitis Media

Charles D. Bluestone, M.D.

Adenoidectomy performed either separately or in combination with tonsillectomy is the most common major surgical procedure employed to prevent otitis media; myringotomy with tympanostomy tube insertion is the most common minor surgical procedure for otitis media with effusion (1).

Tonsil and adenoid surgery are the most common major operations performed in the United States; approximately one-fourth of all children are subjected to tonsillectomy and adenoidectomy during childhood. Such operations account for about one-half of all major surgical operations performed on children, one-fourth of all hospital admissions of children, and 10% of hospital bed-days utilized by children. In 1979, about 634,000 procedures on the tonsils and adenoids were performed in the United States (2), which as shown in Figure 4.1, represents a significant reduction from the over one million such operations performed 10 years earlier.

However, this decrease in the total number of tonsil and adnoid operations may be related to a change in demography, since the total reduction during the same period in the number of children in the age group concerned was approximately 20%. Although the number of adenoidectomies without tonsillectomy remained relatively small in comparison to the number of tonsillectomies either performed separately or in combination with adenoidectomy, there was more than a two-fold increase in the performance of adenoidectomy without tonsillectomy. Also, there appears to be a wide variation in the rate of performance of these operations by region of the country; the rates for adenoidectomy vary the most widely (3). However, there are no data available related to the indications for which these operations were performed. Certainly, for many, otitis media was one of the indications, and in many instances the only indication, for adenoidectomy either with or without tonsillectomy.

PREVIOUS CLINICAL TRIALS

Despite the high frequency of their performance, it has never been established through controlled scientific studies that the benefits of tonsil and adenoid surgery for otitis media exceed their cost in any age group of children. In the past, there have been only a few prospective clinical trials of tonsillectomy and adenoidectomy. The following is a summary of the results of these studies as they relate to the efficacy of the surgical procedures for prevention of otitis media. In 1930, Kaiser (4) reported the results of following 4,400 children, one-half of whom had tonsillectomy and adenoidectomy operations performed (the indications for surgery were not reported). Table 4.1 shows the results of his retrospective analysis of the prevalence of purulent otorrhea 10 years after surgery. Even though there was no difference in incidence of purulent otorrhea in the operated and unoperated children, the study cannot be considered to indicate conclusively the lack of efficacy of tonsillectomy and adenoidectomy in preventing otitis media since: 1) the two groups may not have been similar at the outset; 2) they were not randomized; 3) the analysis was retrospective; and 4) only purulent otor-

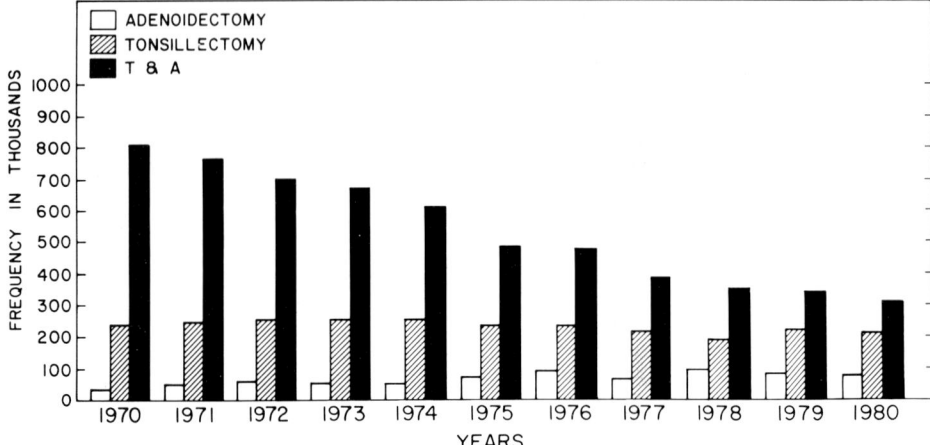

Figure 4.1. Frequency of tonsillectomies and adenoidectomies in all United States nonfederal, short-term hospitals. Estimated in the Ament Hospital Record Study, 1980 (2).

Table 4.1
Prevalence of Purulent Otorrhea in 2,200 Children Who Received Tonsillectomy with Adenoidectomy (T & A) and 2,200 "Comparable" Children Who Did Not (4)

	T & A	No T & A
Before operation	15	12
10 years after operation	5	6

Table 4.2
Mean Incidence of Ititis Media in Children Aged 2–15 Years Receiving Tonsillectomy With Adenoidectomy (T & A) Compared With Control Group (5)

	Control (No.)	T & A (No.)	t
First year	0.33 (154)	0.17 (222)	2.52*
Second year	0.17 (139)	0.14 (213)	0.54

* Significant change $P < .01$

rhea was considered as a measurement of the effectiveness of tonsillectomy and adenoidectomy.

The first truly prospective clinical trial of tonsillectomy and adenoidectomy was reported by McKee (5). The criterion for entry into the study was a history of at least three episodes of "throat infection", or of acute upper respiratory tract infection with cervical adenitis, during the preceding year. Table 4.2 shows the mean incidence of otitis media 1 and 2 years after treatment, in those (randomly chosen) children who underwent tonsillectomy and adenoidectomy compared with those who did not.

The mean incidence of otitis media among control subjects was twice as high as among children having the tonsillectomy and adenoidectomy during the first year of the trial but during the second year, there was no difference in incidence of otitis media in the operated and control groups. However, this study was based on the occurrence of sore throats, and not on the presence of middle ear disease in the year preceding the study. In fact, subjects were initially excluded from the study if they had "marked deafness, or recurrent or chronic otitis media." In addition, the follow-up evaluation was based solely on interview data, with no objective examinations being made, and no attempt was made to detect asymptomatic otitis media with effusion or impairment of hearing.

In a second study, McKee (6) attempted to distinguish the effects of tonsillectomy from those of adenoidectomy. The criterion for entry into the study was the same as in the first study and again, children with deafness and otitis media were excluded. Two hundred children were randomly assigned to undergo either tonsillectomy and adenoidectomy, or adenoidectomy only. Table 4.3 shows that the mean incidence of otitis media in each of the two surgical groups was approximately the same.

Therefore, McKee concluded from the two studies that otitis media was infrequent after adenoidectomy or tonsillectomy and adenoidectomy, and that the combined operation did not offer any particular advantages in the prevention of the disease. Even though the studies did not select children with a high morbidity of otitis media, McKee stated that it was reasonable to infer that adenoidectomy without tonsillectomy was indicated for the prevention of otitis media with effusion.

In 1967, Mawson and coworkers (7) reported their prospective study of tonsillectomy and adenoidectomy. The design of their experiment was similar to that of the first McKee study in that an unspecified number of children who were severely affected were excluded and operated upon. Minimal criteria for entry were not described. Table 4.4 shows the relative incidence of earache and otitis media before, and one and two years after, randomization of 404 children into either the tonsillectomy and adenoidectomy or control group.

There was no apparent difference at any age between the two groups. However, as can be seen from Table 4.4, over one-half of the children apparently did not have otitis media prior to entry and the occurrence of asymptomatic otitis media with effusion or the incidence of hearing loss was not reported.

In a study from New Zealand, using an experimental design similar to McKee's, Roydhouse (8) reported his findings in 1970. In addition to the group of children who were referred for tonsillectomy and adnoidectomy and who were randomized into surgical and no-surgery groups, a third matched group of children who were presumably normal were followed during the trial. Table 4.5 shows the mean incidence of otitis media in the three groups: tonsillectomy and adenoidectomy, tonsillectomy and adenoidectomy withheld, and controls. The results were similar to those reported by McKee, in that there was a reduction in the incidence of otitis media in the first year after tonsillectomy and adenoidectomy but this difference was not maintained into the second year. However, in the second year of the trial, the total duration of otitis media in the tonsillectomy and adenoidectomy group lasted less than 60% as long as they had before surgery. Roydhouse concluded that the operation not only reduced the incidence of otitis media quickly in the first year, but also reduced the severity in both years. However, like the previous studies, patients whose main symptoms were aural were excluded and there was no attempt to detect asymptomatic otitis media with effusion or impairment in hearing. In a second clinical trial, Roydhouse (9) randomly divided 100 children with persistent otitis media into two groups, adenoidectomy with tympanostomy tube insertion and tympanostomy tube insertion alone. All had failed a nonsurgical treatment regimen. He compared these two groups to a third group of 69 other children who had had otitis media but all had been found to be free of middle ear effusion following the nonsurgical measurement and received no surgical treatment.

The cure rate was similar in each of the operative groups with a greater relapse rate in the nonadenoidectomy group, who required 9% more tympanostomy tube insertions. An estimation from radiographs of the size of the adenoids showed that the group cured without surgery had some-

Table 4.3
Incidence and Duration of Otitis Media in Children Aged 2-5 Receiving Tonsillectomy With Adenoidectomy (T & A) or Adenoidectomy (A) Only (6)

	Operation		t
	A	T & A	
No. of Children	97	98	
No. of episodes (per year)	0.16	0.22	0.84
Mean Duration (days per year)	0.55	0.74	0.61

Table 4.4
Relative Frequency Incidence of Earache and Otitis Media in 404 Children Receiving Tonsillectomy with Adenoidectomy (T & A) Compared with Control Group (7)

Number of Episodes	Relative Frequency					
	Year Prior to Trial		1st Year of Trial		2nd Year of Trial	
	T & A %	Control %	T & A %	Control %	T & A %	Control %
0	63	65	59	57	58.5	57.5
1	5	4.5	7.5	15	7	9.5
2–3	19	22.5	15.5	18	9	11
4–6	6	3	3.5	2	1	1.5
>7	5	4		2.5		1

Table 4.5
Mean Incidence per Year of Otitis Media in Children Receiving Tonsillectomy with Adenoidectomy (T & A) Compared with Two Control Groups (8)

	T & A (No.)	T & A Withheld (No.)	Control (No.)
1st Year of Trial	0.19 (251)	0.29 (175)	0.12 (173)
2nd Year of Trial	0.09 (204)	0.07 (122)	0.08 (173)

what smaller adenoids. The relapse rate in the nonadenoidectomy surgical group was independent of the size of the adenoids. The study failed to show a favorable outcome following adenoidectomy.

Unfortunately, all of these prospective controlled studies had one or more of the following limitations in experimental design: 1) entry into the study was based on the occurrence of a sore throat and not on the presence of otitis media; 2) objective evidence of otitis media was not documented by tympanometry or audiometry; 3) no other srgical procedures which may have been performed (myringotomy or tympanostomy tube insertions, for example) were reported; 4) the technique of adenoidectomy—e.g., "mid-line sweep" or thorough removal of adenoid tissue from the fossa of Rosenmüller—was not described, nor was evidence of complete removal of the adenoids documented; and 5) nasal and Eustachian tube function were not assessed objectively.

CHILDREN'S HOSPITAL OF PITTSBURGH STUDY

At the Children's Hospital of Pittsburgh, a prospective controlled study is currently in progress to determine the efficacy of tonsillectomy and adenoidectomy. The effect of adenoidectomy on otitis media with effusion is one of the primary research questions, and an attempt is being made to document and control those factors cited as lacking in the previous studies cited above. The criterion for entry into the study (to deal with the adenoidectomy-for-otitis media with effusion problem) is documented episodes of recurrent or persistent otitis media with effusion in a child who had had a myringotomy and insertion of a tympanostomy tube at least once previously. Applying stringent surgical indications, of course, requires careful evaluation. After initial examination, each patient is examined every 6 weeks and at the time of any respiratory illness. Pneumatic otoscopy is always performed at every visit. A trained interviewer telephones each home every 2 weeks to determine whether there had been apparent or suspected illness, to make sure that any ill child is brought in promptly for examination, and to obtain routine information on school attendance, medication usage, and a number of minor symptoms.

Basic allergy screening is part of every

child's work-up. A nasal smear is examined for eosinophiles, and a battery of skin tests using common inhalant allergens is applied. Other regularly performed studies include lateral soft tissue radiographs of the nasopharynx, to assess adenoid size; sinus radiographs, when sinusitis is suspected; and audiometry and tympanometry, to evaluate hearing and middle ear status and tympanic membrane compliance.

The degree of middle ear disease developing in the adenoidectomy and nonadenoidectomy groups, respectively, is measured on the basis of three main parameters: 1) number of episodes per year of otitis media with effusion; 2) months of middle ear effusion; and 3) frequency with which myringotomy is carried out subsequent to entering the clinical trial.

Data concerning subjects assigned randomly either to receive adenoidectomy or to enter the nonadenoidectomy control group are maintained separately from data concerning subjects whose parents decline randomization and opt for or against adenoidectomy. However, the two groups of data appear similar.

Preliminary analyses of data currently available may be summarized by stating that, in study subjects: 1) adenoidectomy by no means eliminates the problem of recurrent otitis media, and 2) it remains at the present time uncertain whether or not adenoidectomy somewhat reduces the rate, severity, or duration of recurrent episodes (10). The following variables are being examined as potentially important in affecting the outcome of adenoidectomy for otitis media with effusion: age, sex, race, allergy, adenoid size, and Eustachian tube function.

This study does not address the question of whether tonsillectomy and adenoidectomy is more effective in the prevention of otitis media with effusion than adenoidectomy alone, nor will it answer the question of the relative value of adenoidectomy with or without tonsillectomy for children who have not received myringotomy and insertion of tympanostomy tubes in the past. These questions are being addressed at present in a randomized clinical trial currently being conducted at the same institution.

EFFECT OF ADENOIDECTOMY ON EUSTACHIAN TUBE FUNCTION

In an attempt to improve criteria for the preoperative selection of patients for adenoidectomy, radiographic studies of the nasopharynx and Eustachian tube prior to surgery and after adenoidectomy were reported (11). Of 27 patients who had preoperative obstruction of the nasophryngeal end of the Eustachian tube, adenoidectomy appeared to be helpful in 19 (70%). Results appeared to be quite poor in children with nasal allergy: only 2 of 10 had good results. Furthermore, children who had preopertively show reflux of contrast medium from the nasopharynx into the middle ear did not benefit from adenoidectomy. In this study, 20 of 33 children (60%) seemed to have a favorable response to adenoidectomy but 8 had worse middle ear disease after the operation than before. For example, a few of the children who had asymptomatic otitis media with effusion prior to adenoidectomy developed recurrent acute symptomatic otitis media with effusion following the procedure. Figure 4.2 shows an example of a lateral roentgenographic study of a child with chronic secretory otitis media who received an adenoidectomy. Before surgery, the adenoids were adjudged to be of only moderate size. Eight weeks following the adenoidectomy, the adenoid size appeared only somewhat smaller. However, when the pre- and postadenoidectomy submental-vertex views were compared in the same child, the function of the Eustachian tube at the nasopharyngeal end appeared obstructed before the operation and normal following the operation (Fig. 4.3). This example demonstrates that lateral roentgenographic views alone may not be sufficient to assess the effect of the adnoids on the nasopharyngeal end of the Eustachian tube.

The ventilatory function of the Eustachian tube has been studied using the inflation-deflation manometric technique

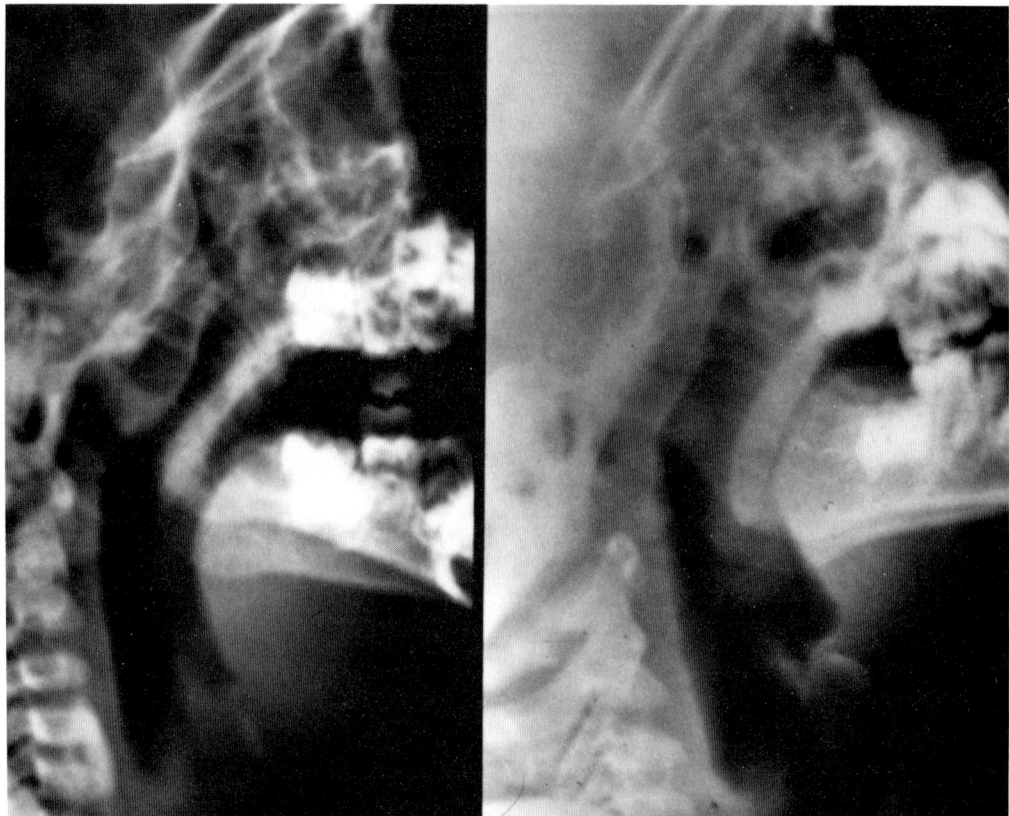

Figure 4.2. Lateral roentgenograms of the soft tissue of the head and neck of a child with chronic otitis media with effusion. Prior to adenoidectomy the adenoids were considered to be of only moderate size (*left*). Postadenoidectomy they appeared slightly smaller (*right*).

both before and after adenoidectomy in a group of children with otitis media with effusion in whom a tympanostomy tube had been inserted (12). Inflation-deflation studies of the Eustachian tube were obtained in ears that remained intubated, aerated, and dry both before and 8 weeks after adenoidectomy. Nasal pressures during swallowing were also determined in some. The results of this study indicated that, following adenoidectomy, Eustachian tube ventilatory function improved in some, remained the same in others, and in a few children, the function appeared to have been made worse. Improvement was related to a reduction of extrinsic mechanical obstruction of the Eustachian tube (Fig. 4.4), or to nasal obstruction due to the adenoids (Fig. 4.5), while in those in whom the function was adjudged worse the tube was considered to be more pliant after the adenoidectomy than before. This increase in compliance was attributed to loss of adenoid support of the Eustachian tube in the fossa of Rosenmüller (Fig. 4.6). A comparable situation was described in the radiographic study in which several of the children demonstrated reflux of radiopaque liquid medium from the nasopharynx into the middle ear after the adenoidectomy but not before (Fig. 4.7).

However, neither of these studies included control subjects. In the current study tonsillectomy and adenoidectomy

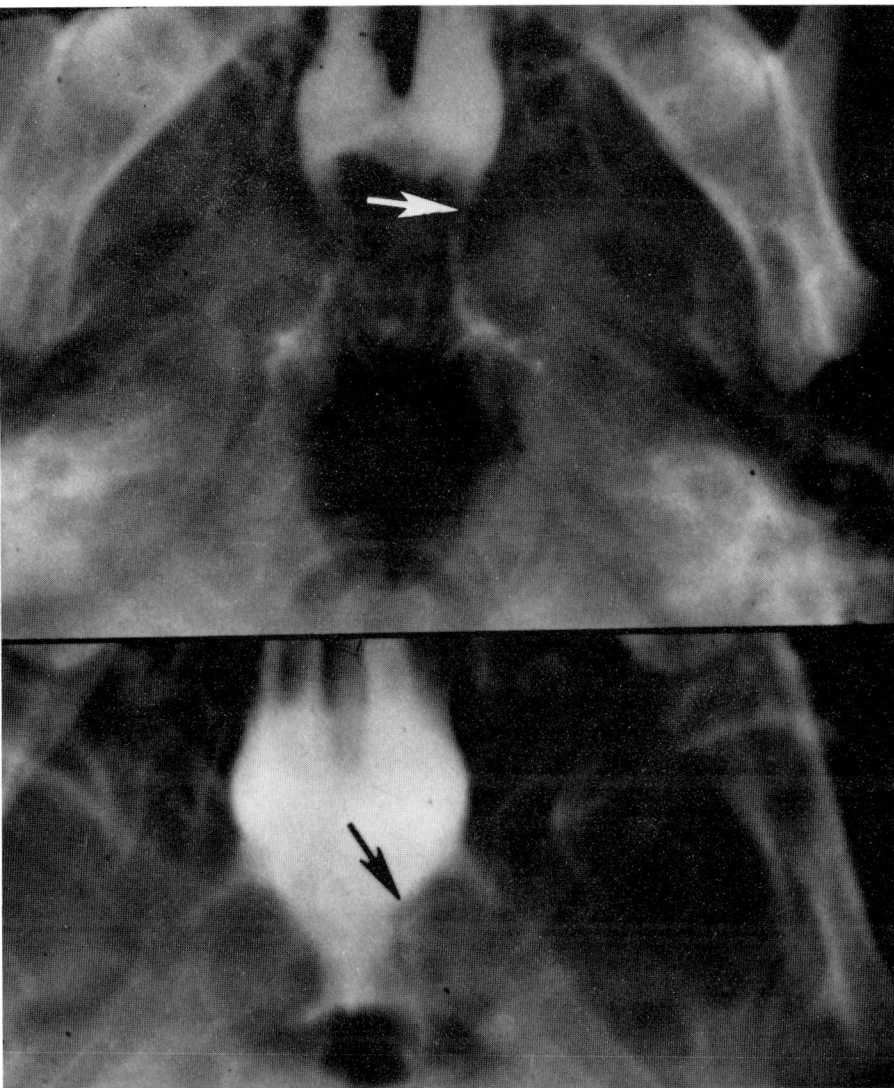

Figure 4.3. Preadenoidectomy submental-vertex roentgenogram (*top*) demonstrating extrinsic compression of the nasopharyngeal end of the Eustachian tube (*arrow*) in the same child described in Figure 4.2. Following adenoidectomy (*bottom*), contrast material entered the mouth of the Eustachian tube and the torus tubarius (*arrow*) was not obstructed by the adenoids.

being conducted at the Children's Hospital of Pittsburgh, Eustachian tube ventilatory function studies employing the inflation-deflation manometric technique are performed prior to and after randomized selection of children for the study and at any time an upper respiratory tract infection supervenes. Since Eustachian tube ventilatory function has been shown to be affected adversely by an upper respiratory tract infection (13), it is important to assess this function when an upper respiratory tract infection is present as well as when infection is absent in children both before

28 Clinical Otology

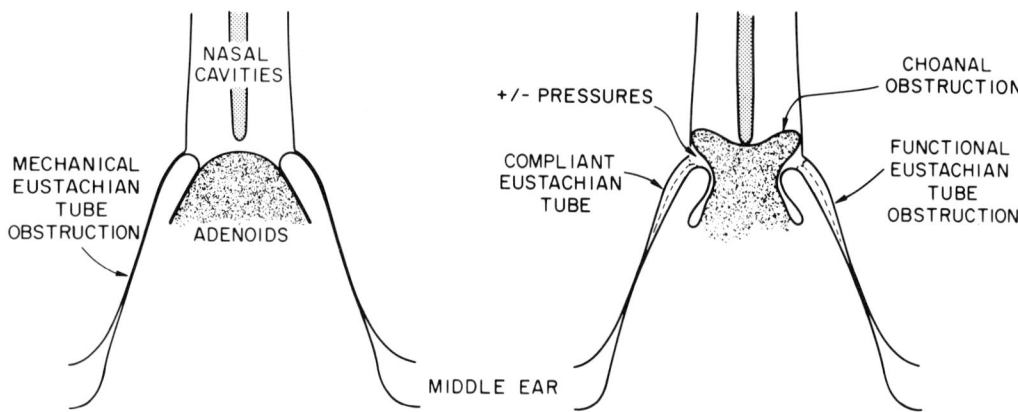

Figure 4.4. Two proposed mechanisms by which obstructive adenoids could alter Eustachian tube function. The adenoids can cause extrinsic mechanical compression of the Eustachian tube in the fossa of Rosenmüller (*left*). Obstruction of the posterior nasal choanae may result in abnormal nasopharyngeal pressures that develop during swallowing (Toynbee phenomenon) and result in either insufflation into the middle ear of nasopharyngeal secretions or prevent the tube from opening, or both (*right*).

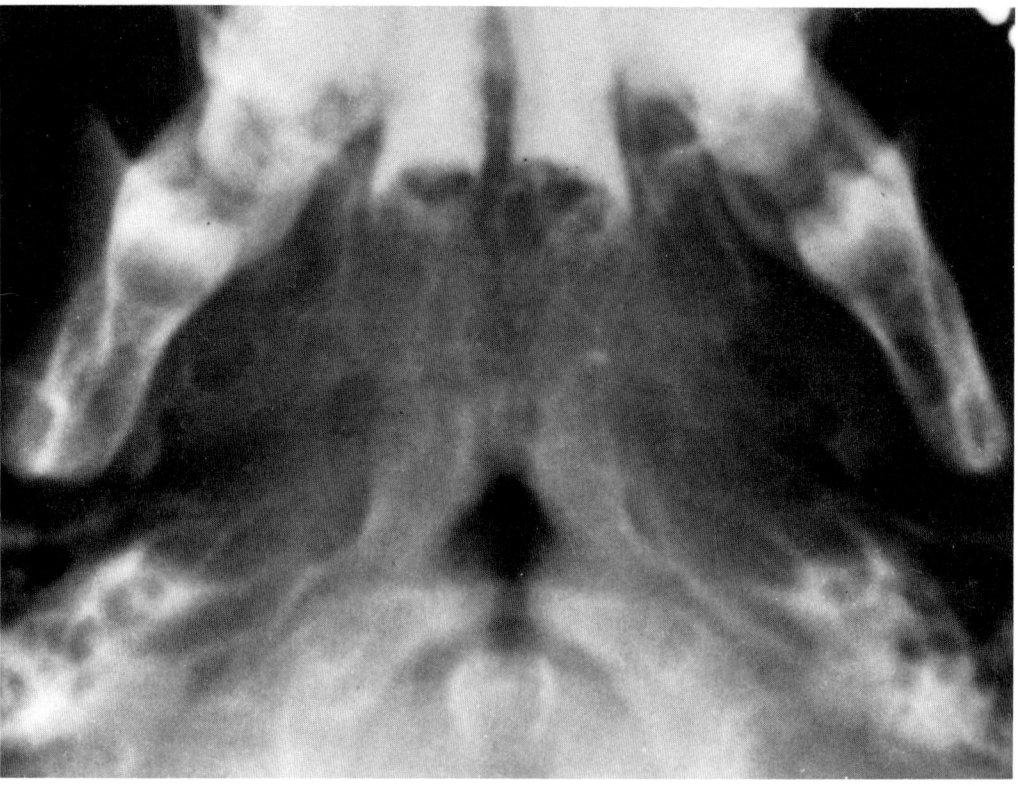

Figure 4.5. Submental-vertex roentgenogram of a child with adenoids obstructing the posterior nasal choanae.

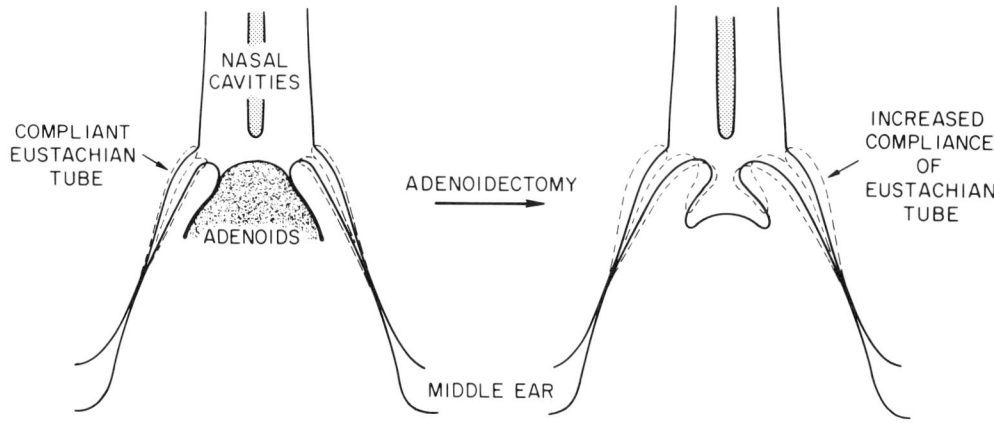

Figure 4.6. Proposed mechanism by which removal of adenoids can result in more pliant Eustachian tube after surgery than before. The increase in compliance following the surgery may be due to decrease in tubal support as a result of the adenoids being removed from the fossa of Rosenmüller.

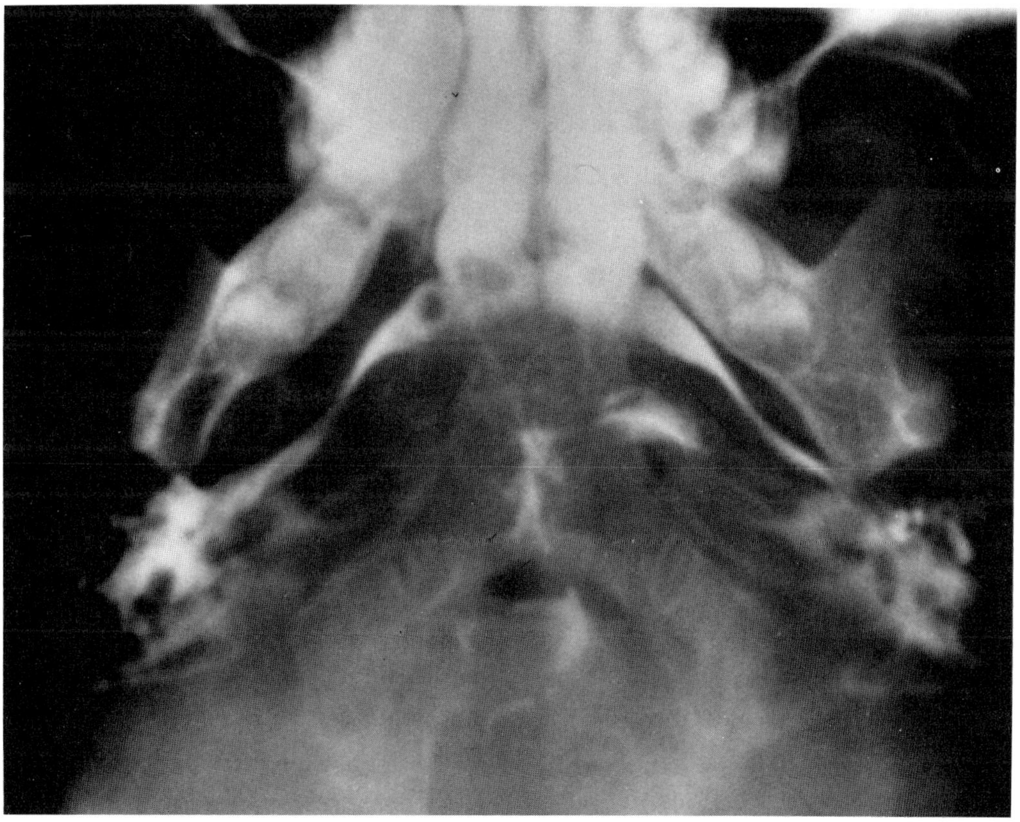

Figure 4.7. Postadenoidectomy radiograph of a child who demonstrated reflux of radiopaque media from the nasopharynx into the middle ear. This did not occur during the preadenoidectomy radiographic study.

and after randomization into either the adenoidectomy or control group. The goal of this study is to determine if adenoidectomy is efficacious in preventing otitis media with effusion in children, and if so, whether or not a simple Eustachian tube function test may be helpful in determining who may be helped by the procedure. An additional question would be which type of adenoidectomy (mid-line sweep or also removing the adenoids from the fossa of Rosenmüller) is indicated for the individual child. Hopefully, some or all of these questions will be answered by the current studies.

CONCLUSIONS

The previous prospective studies to determine the efficacy of tonsillectomy and adenoidectomy or adenoidectomy for otitis media have shown a modest reduction in the incidence of ear disease in some studies (5, 6, 8) but no reduction in others (4, 7, 9) following surgery. However, all of these studies, unfortunately, suffered from shortcomings in design and method. The current studies of tonsillectomy and adenoidectomy being conducted in Pittsburgh are attempting to eliminate the problems of the earlier studies and to answer the question of whether adenoidectomy is helpful in decreasing otitis media, so that children who stand to benefit can be helped while those who may not can be spared the cost, discomfrot, and risks of surgery.

References

1. Paradise, J.L. On tympanostomy tubes, rationale, results, reservations, and recommendations. Pediatrics 60: 86–90, 1977.
2. Ament, R.P. Hospital Record Study, Professional Activity Study. Commission on Professional and Hospital Activities, Ann Arbor, Michigan, 1980.
3. National Center for Health Statistics. Surgical Operations in Short-Stay Hospitals: United States—1971. (DHEW Publication No. HRA-75-1769), United States Department of Health, Education and Welfare, Rockville, MD., 1974.
4. Kaiser, A.D. Results on tonsillectomy: A comparative study of 2,200 tonsillectomized children with an equal number of controls three and ten years after operation. JAMA 95: 837–842, 1930.
5. McKee, W.J.E. A controlled study of the effects of tonsillectomy and adenoidectomy in children. Br J Prev Soc Med 17: 46–49, 1963.
6. McKee, W.J.E. The part played by adenoidectomy in the combined operation of tonsillectomy with adenoidectomy: Second part of a controlled study in children. Br J Prev Soc Med 17: 133–140, 1963.
7. Mawson, S.R., Adlington, R., and Evans, M. A controlled study evaluation of adeno-tonsillectomy in children. J Laryngol Otol 81: 777–790, 1967.
8. Roydhouse, N. A controlled study of adeno-tonsillectomy. Arch Otolaryngol 92: 611–616, 1970.
9. Roydhouse, N. Adenoidectomy for otitis media with effusion. Ann Otol Rhinol Laryngol 89 (Suppl. 68): 312–315, 1980.
10. Paradise, J.L., Bluestone, C.D., Rodgers, K.D., and Taylor, F.H. Efficacy of adenoidectomy in recurrent otitis media: Historical overview and preliminary results from a randomized, controlled trial. Ann Otol Rhinol Laryngol 89 (Suppl. 68): 319–321, 1980.
11. Bluestone, C.D., Wittel, R.A., Paradise, J.L. et al. Eustachian tube function as related to adenoidectomy for otitis media. Trans Am Acad Ophthalmol Otolaryngol 76: 1325–1339, 1972.
12. Bluestone, C.D., Cantekin, E.I., and Beery, Q.C. Certain effects of adenoidectomy on Eustachian tube ventilatory function. Laryngoscope 85: 113–127, 1975.
13. Bluestone, C.D., Cantekin, E.I., and Beery, Q.C. Effect of inflammation on the ventilatory function of the Eustachian tube. Laryngoscope 87: 493–507, 1977.

CHAPTER 5

Tympanosclerosis Cause and Prevention

Maurice Schiff, M.D.

The prevention of tympanosclerosis must take place 20 to 30 years before it becomes manifest or apparent. The major health professionals involved at this stage are the general practitioner and the pediatrician. The otologist does not become involved until the disease has progressed to a sufficient stage as to cause either the symptoms of discharge or the insidious onset of hearing loss.

The episodes of acute otitis media are usually seen by the family physician and/or pediatrician. If the disease is in the chronic stage, the child may be referred to an otologist. In the early stages, it should be possible to somewhat determine by good visualization of the tympanic membrane the nature of the process going on. Having a child with serious otitis media where one can see the amber, or clear, fluid from the other side of the drum permits a conservative handling of the problem depending upon the etiologic factors involved. If the causative organism is streptococcus, hemophilus influenzae, or pneumococcus, this should sound a red alert to the possibility of developing suppuration in the middle ear. The visualization of a drum that is so thick and turgescent that no amount of transparency exists, together with even a small degree of bulging, should make one start to think of the necessity of draining this ear.

The general surgical principle of draining abscesses is well documented in all other parts of the anatomy, so why should this not be true for the middle ear. The desire to be conservative at this point can

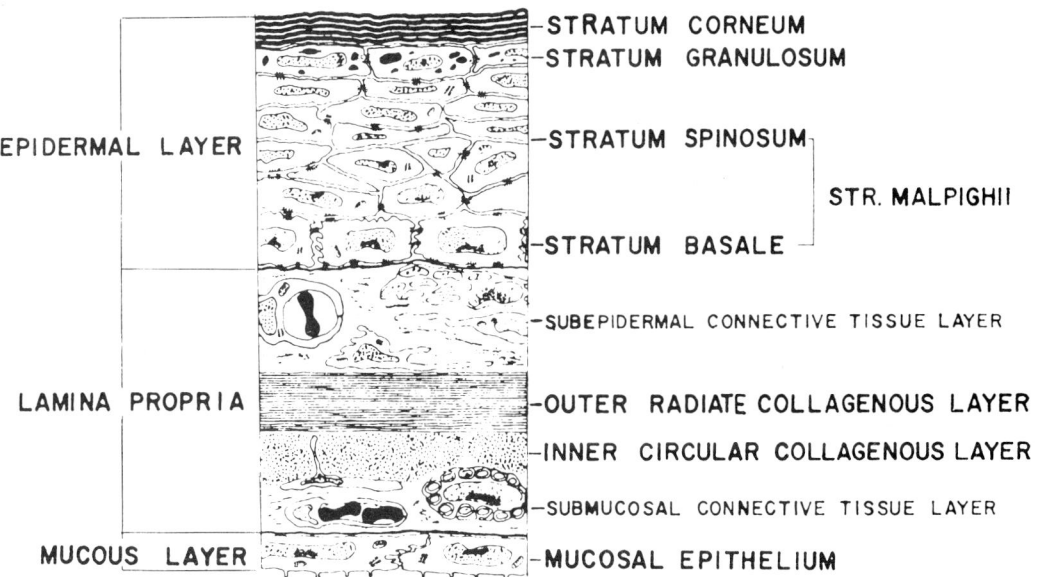

Figure 5.1.

now be viewed as radical. The fact that a large number of these infections produce suppuration in the middle ear despite the presence of antibiotics should be noted. In many cases, the suppuration becomes sterile pus after the antibiotic levels have achieved a high enough concentration. Usually it is difficult to get antibiotics into pus spaces. Once the pus has ruptured the eardrum, the process thereby initiated is capable of starting tympanosclerosis. That is not to say that all drums that rupture in fact will develop tympanosclerosis. To the contrary, only a small percentage of them do this depending upon the nature and the amount of damage involved.

In order to rupture the drum, the tympanic membrane has to undergo a local area of necrosis in which there is, indeed, a loss of vascular supply and a necrotic ischemic death of the tissue which is about to give way. In this process, one can easily visualize the local damage and degradation of the various layers of the tympanic membrane by the necrosis. Locally degenerated products are reabsorbed and function as stimuli for local antibody formation against these foreign protein antigens. These antigens are part of what was once the eardrum recognized as "self" but now, having been necrotized, are broken into components identified as "other." The best

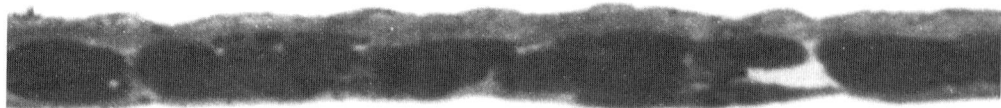

Figure 5.2.

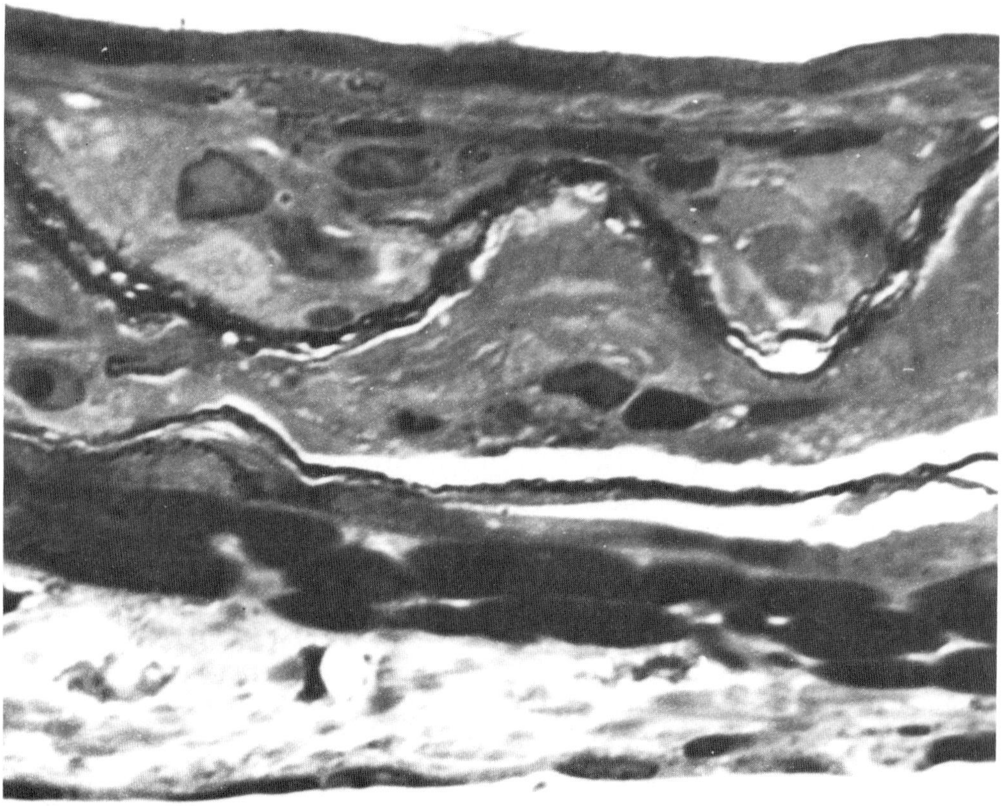

Figure 5.3.

example of this can be seen most frequently in those ears that have had scarlatina with otitis media. The loss of the eardrum is huge leading to subtotal perforation. In former years, before the era of tympanoplasty, these people grew up to adulthood having almost uniformly areas of tympanosclerosis in the margins of the remaining portion of the tympanic membrane extending to the annulus tympanicus.

Hemophilus, likewise, has the capacity to create an enormously disproportionate amount of edema considering the amount of infection. With this edema, the ground substance of the inner and middle layers of the tympanic membrane now become permeable to substances which were formerly kept out. As local ischemia takes place, the autolytic processes break down the various protein components which now, again, become the sensitizing antigens to initiate the process for tympanosclerosis.

The first infection is almost never the cause of tympanosclerosis. This is the sensitizing infection. The subsequent challenging infections either increase the sensitivity of the area by repeated antigen stimulation or set about to challenge that which has already been set up in the middle ear and tympanic membrane. Since tympanosclerosis is essentially a disease of the middle layer of the drum and of the lamina propria of the middle ear, it is important to consider the requirement of an antigen to be able to arrive at this layer to produce its sensitizing reaction.

PATHOGENESIS

To clarify this point, in Figure 5.1 one can see the cross section of the tympanic membrane of the pars tensa of the squirrel monkey. Particular attention should be paid to the lamina propria layer. Figure 5.2 shows the normal tympanic membrane of the guinea pig with the three layers easily

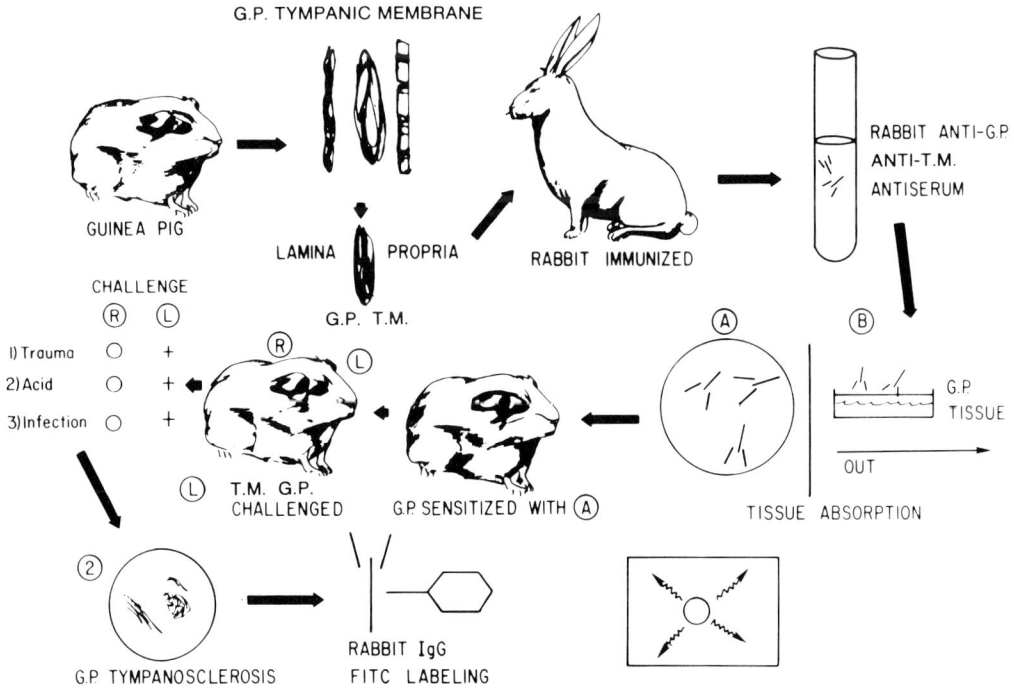

EXPERIMENTAL TYMPANOSCLEROSIS

Figure 5.4.

identified at ×400 magnification. The loose layer of subepidermal connective tissue contributes minimally to the thickness of the drum. Figure 5.3 is the picture of the guinea pig whose body has been sensitized with the proper antitympanic membrane material, and now the drum is challenged. This dark band of calcification has occurred in less than 90 days in the subepithelial connective tissue layer. Note how thick this layer is. The submucosal connective tissue layer is so thick that it would require extending the slide several inches more to finally reach the mucosal epithelium. This is at the same magnification ×400.

Figure 5.4 shows the model that was used to develop this animal experimental tympanosclerosis. It is almost 250 years since Cassebohm (1) in 1734 described conditions which later became recognized and identified as tympanosclerosis. Since that time, many experimental methods have been tried to produce this disease entity without success. Not only does this method permit visualization of the development of tympanosclerosis, but this is also detectable using fluorescent antibody techniques which means that what we have produced is quite specific for the antiguinea pig antitympanic antibodies. Further confirmation can be better visualized in the electron micrograph of the tympanic membrane in Figure 5.5 and the induced one in Figure 5.6 with tympanosclerosis, both ×8000. Not only is the mitochondria visualized, but the calcification of the mitochondria, which has been seen previously in specimens of human tympanosclerosis by Chang (2), can also be noted. With the calcification of the mitochondria, one can immediately speculate

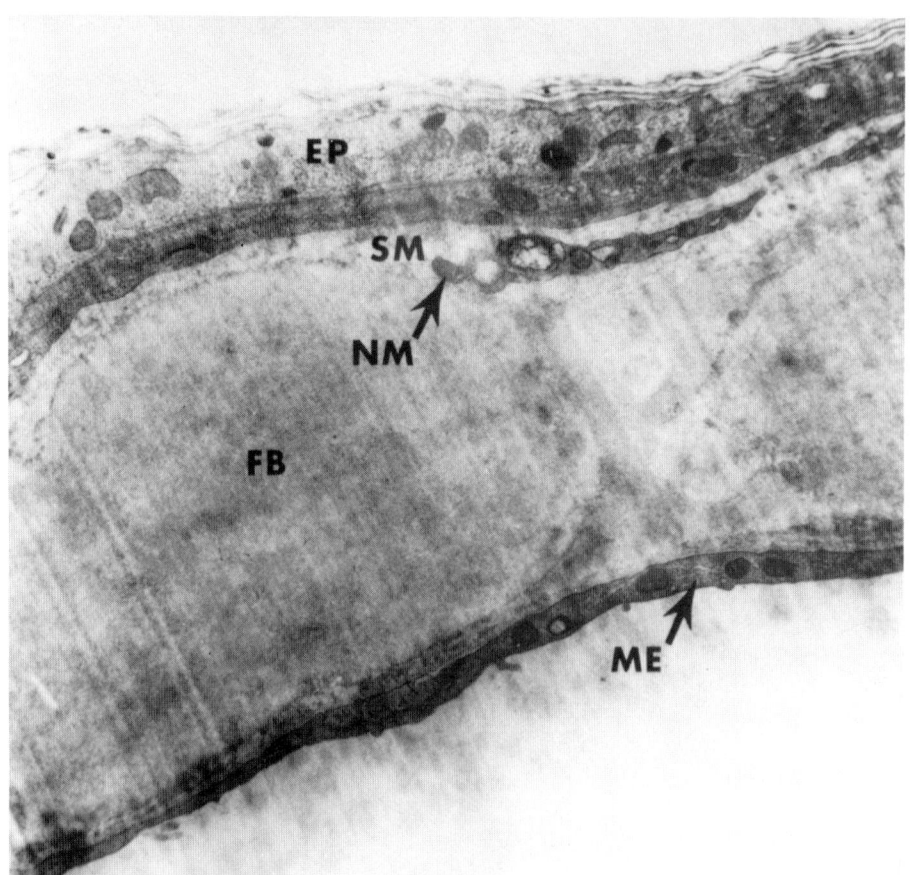

Figure 5.5.

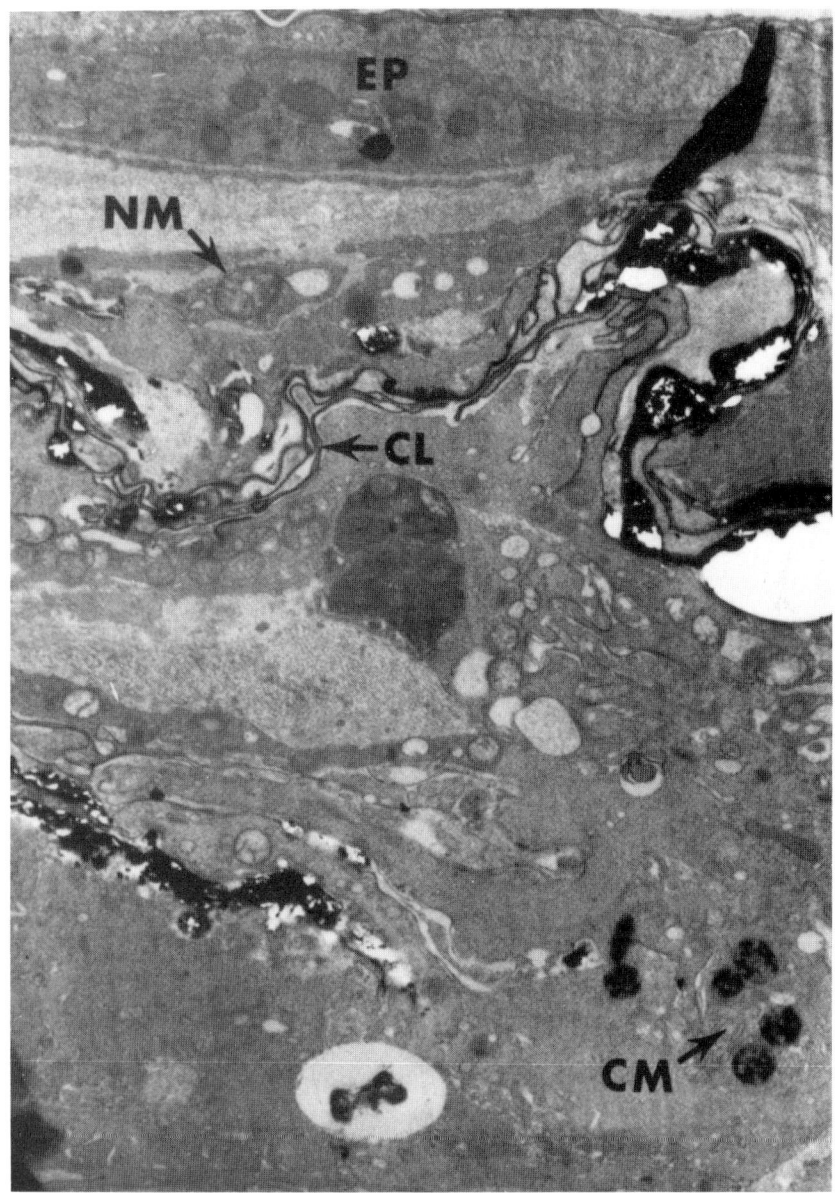

Figure 5.6.

on the changes in the oxidation capabilities of the damaged tissues. This deposition of calcium within the mitochondria is caused by changes within the mitochondria itself rather than saturation from blood calcium.

The question as to why ears with tympanosclerosis and perforation are so often dry can be better answered in light of the work of Tos and Bak-Pedersen (3) who showed that as the disease progresses, the activity of the mucus glands per se is decreased considerably and is slowly practically eliminated.

The query is often made as to why don't all of the ears resolve to a normal state, or why don't they all develop tympanosclerosis? Figure 5.7 shows the hypothetical diagram which is proposed to the regulation of the laying down of collagen and its removal. As with most infections, there is a stimulation of the fibroblast to elaborate

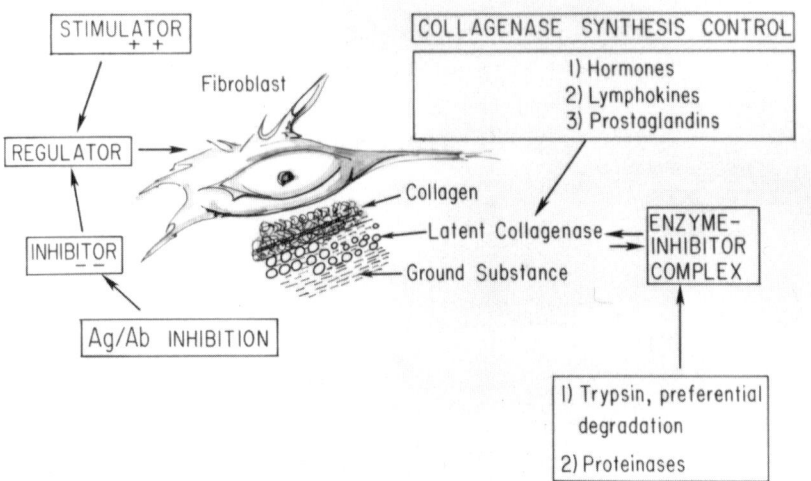

Figure 5.7.

more collagen, and this is acted upon by regulators. Likewise, in this situation, it would appear that the inhibitor is being inhibited, or neutralized, by this antigen antibody reaction process permitting an excessive amount of collagen to be elaborated. This would explain the excess of the deposit. Why this is not absorbed and degraded like most other ear infections is best understood in looking at the latent collagenase which apparently is not permitted to act on the collagen in degrading it for removal. A more elaborate understanding of this is in Figure 5.8 which is from the excellent monograph by Perez-Tamayo (4) on the degradation of collagen. If there is either excessive laying down, or failure to resculpture and reabosrb the degraded collagen, you have the essence of most dense scar tissue formation. Each block of this diagram is an excellent subject for discussion and has bearing on wound healing and tissue repair in general.

THE CLINICAL TYMPANOSCLEROSIS

In Kinney's excellent paper (5), he noted that there was a 20% incidence of some form of tympanosclerosis in almost 1500 chronic ear surgeries reviewed. Of these, 80% were over the age of 30; 78% had histories of over 10 years duration, and 20% had histories of 6 months to 10 years duration. Only 2% had a history of less than 6 months duration. Of these patients, 66% had dry ears, and 33% had mucoid or purulent discharge.

It should be of considerable clinical interest that in an ear with tympanosclerosis that has discharge, one should be suspicious of coexistence of cholesteatoma. Statistics would seem to indicate that this is really not a cause and effect but a simple coexistence.

Ossicular chain fixation may take place by hyalinized collagen, new bone growth, or fibrous tissue as noted by Schuknecht (6). The attention to pseudo-otosclerosis, or fixation of the ossicular chain, for other reasons than classic otosclerosis was amplified and clarified by Goodhill (7).

Thus, we have a clinical entity that starts in childhood, is curable and preventable in childhood, and makes its manifestation in adulthood. Both Nager (8) and Kinney (5) also emphasized the requirement of early diagnosis and treatment. The further emphasis on prevention, now that a theory of pathogenesis is tenable, is a valuable adjunct in the treatment of a disease before it occurs.

REGULATION OF COLLAGEN DEGRADATION

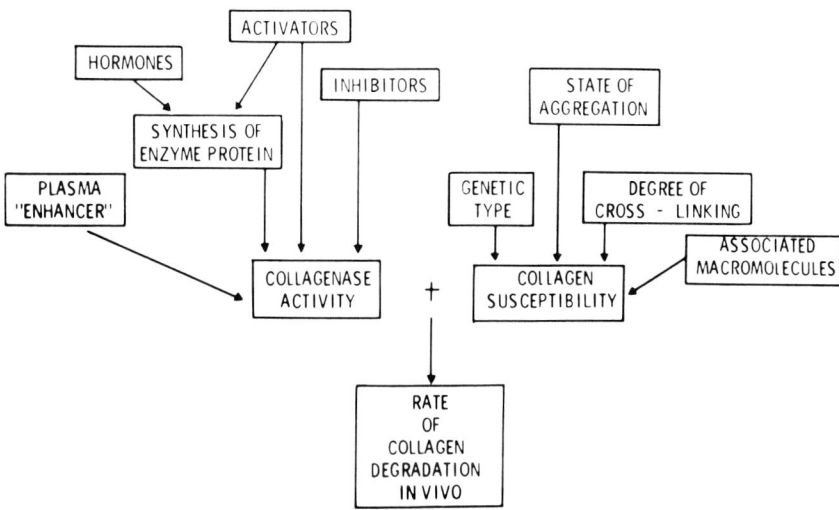

Figure 5.8.

To this end, it becomes a requirement of the otologic community to promulgate this type of information to our general practitioner and pediatric colleagues. In the second half of the 20th century, the greatest emphasis in medicine has been laid in prevention. This is based and grounded on better understanding of cause and effect. It would appear that as otologists we might be able to put ourselves out of tympanosclerosis business by proper preventive education.

References

1. Cassebohm, I.F. Tractatus quatuor anatomici de aure humana, 1734.
2. Chang, I.W. Tympanosclerosis. Electron microscopic study. *Acta Otolaryngol (Stockh)* 68: 62–72, 1969.
3. Tos, M., and Bak-Pedersen, K. Middle ear mucosa in tympanosclerosis. *J Laryngol Otol* 88: 119–26, 1974.
4. Perez-Tamayo, R. The pathology of collagen degradation. *Am J Pathol* 92: 508–66, 1979.
5. Kinney, S.E. Postinflammatory ossicular fixation in tympanoplasty. *Laryngoscope* 88: 821–38, 1978.
6. Schuknecht, H. *Pathology of the Ear.* Cambridge, Harvard University Press, 1974.
7. Goodhill, V. Pseudo-otosclerosis. *Laryngoscope* 70: 722–57, 1960.
8. Nager, G.T. Pathology of acute and chronic otitis media and their complications. In *Otitis Media*, Charles C. Thomas, Springfield, IL, pp. 103–123, 1972.

CHAPTER 6

Cholesteatoma Surgery with Obliteration: Late Results

Tauno Palva, M.D.

At the end of 1950's, two new trends in ear surgery became obvious. Both wanted to get rid of the large, open, modified radical mastoid cavities and to end up postoperatively with nearly normal ear canals. Powerful antibiotics, better drills, and the routine use of magnification gave and added sense of security to the new generation of ear surgeons. One school, started by Myers and Schlosser (1), and particularly by Jansen (20), recommended the canal wall up technique which, at one stage, was improperly called intact canal wall procedure. This operation presupposes that total eradication of cholesteatomatous disease can be made notwithstanding the obstacle formed by the canal wall.

The other school of thought was represented by Guilford (3) and myself (4, 5), both of us being convinced by our past surgical experience, that total removal of cholesteatomatous disease cannot be made while the posterior canal wall is up. Without canal wall removal, we could not obtain a satisfactory exposure of the Eustachian tube or remove to our satisfaction the epitympanic extensions of the disease. The conclusion, therefore, was that the surgeon must do a classic modified radical mastoidectomy first, with this unsurpassed exposure eradicate cholesteatomatous disease, and only from this stage start reconstruction of the ear. This has been my continuing line from the late 1950's: I have tried most of the fashion procedures a few times only to return more convinced than ever to the procedure developed during those years.

In this paper, I will report mainly on a series of 411 cholesteatoma ears that were operated upon during 1964–1971, while I was heading the University of Oulu Ear-Nose-Throat (ENT) Department. This is not the best material upon which to report on mastoid obliteration and tympanoplasty because of the operative technique has been improved since this period by adding the routine use of bone paté, bone chips, and lyophilized dura to the obliteration procedure. Moreover, during this period, in addition to the ossicles, we used polythene and stainless steel wire prostheses in reconstruction (6) but after this time, we changed entirely to the use of autograft, homograft, or cortical bone ossicular reconstruction. However, as far as eradication of cholesteatomatous disease goes, the material represents our present technique closely enough to give a reliable picture of the outcome.

Briefly, the essential reconstructive technique at that time was to make a postauricular incision, to create a musculoperiosteal flap, and to do a modified radical mastoidectomy. After reconstruction of the ossicles with various materials, the anterior part of the temporal muscle fascia was used for tympanic membrane reconstruction while the larger posterior part was lifted up to surround the gauze-filled soft ear canal. The musculoperiosteal flap was placed behind this structure; in a limited number of cases, inorganic bone was used to fill the possibly still remaining empty cavity. From 1973 on (7), the improved procedure for obliteration has been in routine use.

Follow-up results of this early material have been reported by us in 1973 (8) and later amplified in a doctoral dissertation by Ojala (9).

SURGICAL METHODS FOR REMOVAL OF CHOLESTEATOMATOUS DISEASE

In my routine surgery, I employ two methods of operations. One is endaural atticotomy which provides access to cholesteatomata that are limited to the tympanic or anterior epitympanic areas, with no disease in the mastoid. These cases range 5-10%, all others receiving the postauricular modified radical surgery approach. The latter is the subject of the following appraisal.

CANAL SIZE AFTER OBLITERATION

We have analyzed the postoperative state of the ear canal in several papers (9, 10) and we measured preoperatively, during surgery, and postoperatively the size of the ear canal, resp. modified radical cavity, with saline. Early postoperatively, the ear canal volume was smaller than preoperatively, but after a period of 3 months, a gradual widening started that continued during the first 3 years. Cavitation of the ear canal was directly related to the measured volume of the operative cavity, and in small and medium sized (<3 ml, 3-7 ml) cavities, the reconstructed ear canal was normal in a large majority of cases or slightly wider than normal. Marked cavitation of ear canal in operative cavities in excess of 7 ml occurred in 47% of cases and in these ears, annual wax removal was necessary similar to original modified radical operation without obliteration.

Another problem that became evident was that the ears developing cavitation were more likely to develop occasional infection especially in ears with a narrow outer entrance. These occurred in 12% of the ears and needed regular care. Contributing causes to the discharge were the use of foreign material (stainless steel, polythene, silastic) in the middle ear and insufficient removal of all tympanic pathologically altered mucosa, or perilabyrinthine cells. Of these ears, 16% had increased numbers of eosinophilic and mast cells in the discharge concomitant with nasal allergy.

When these results were noted in 1973, I advocated the use of bone paté and bone chips for improved obliteration (7, 11), combined with the use of lyophilized dura. Similarly, all foreign material has been discarded including polythene, stainless steel, and silastic sheeting. The latter is used only in narrow areas between the reconstructed ossicles, facial canal, and sometimes in the Eustachian tube in the form of a tongue that keeps the lumen open during epithelialization. All larger raw surfaces are covered by thin pieces of lyophilized dura and only ossicles or cortical bone are used for ossicular reconstruction. The only exception I make as to foreign material is the use of TORP or PORP shaft as a bridge between the footplate, resp. stapes, and an incus body medial to the tympanic membrane (12). In all ears with a narrow ear canal, a meatoplasty is performed to be wide postoperatively.

In the cases since 1974 that I have operated upon following these principles, real cavitation is seen only exceptionally and even then it is generally not larger than a small, open, modified radical cavity in a sclerotic mastoid. In my personal experience, of the last 200 cases operated upon, none shows continuous discharge but in 5%, there is occasional discharge necessitating one to three follow-up visits annually. In 95% of the cases, I recommend the follow-up every 2 or 3 years if the first 3 years have passed without problems.

RECURRENCE OF CHOLESTEATOMA

In this original material of 411 ears from the period 1964-1971, the figure for cholesteatoma recurrence was 4.6% with an average follow-up time of 8.8 years. A more recent analysis with a follow-up time of 12 years has shown recurrent cholesteatoma to have increased to 6%. Considering the long observation time, one can safely conclude that only part of these are residual cholesteatomata and that the late ones have developed due to recurrent infectious disease as a papillary ingrowth. None of the cholesteatomata have developed behind the musculoperiosteal flap in the obliterated cavity and I do not see any possibility of this development if the surgeon is well trained and uses his clinical judgment not to obliterate if in doubt.

In a series of cholesteatoma ears from the Helsinki clinic, operated upon between 1975 and the end of 1979, about 200 cases are presently under analysis, and the figure for recurrent cholesteatoma is less than 4%.

At present, only Smyth (13) has produced figures for residual cholesteatoma using my obliteration approach. In his experience, cholesteatoma was found in a planned second stage surgery in as many as 20% of cases. In his hands, the figures for residual cholesteatoma, using various approaches, are the same in a planned second stage. His residuals were mostly in the mesotympanum and less in the epitympanum. In one case, he had cholesteatoma developing under the flap.

I have wondered why results of this kind can occur in trained hands. In my estimate, the answer lies in the lacking radicality with mucosal removal. More than 15 years ago, I started to take tympanic mucosal biopsies from various areas showing no clinical cholesteatoma (14). To my great surprise, initially, there was squamous migrating epithelium in many areas judged to contain only mucosal edema. My present routine evaluation shows that tympanic biopsies produce histological evidence of squamous epithelium in the areas in 15% which were recorded free in the clinical notes. This would agree quite well with our 5% recurrence as compared with the 20% recurrence in the other series (Figs. 6.1–6.3).

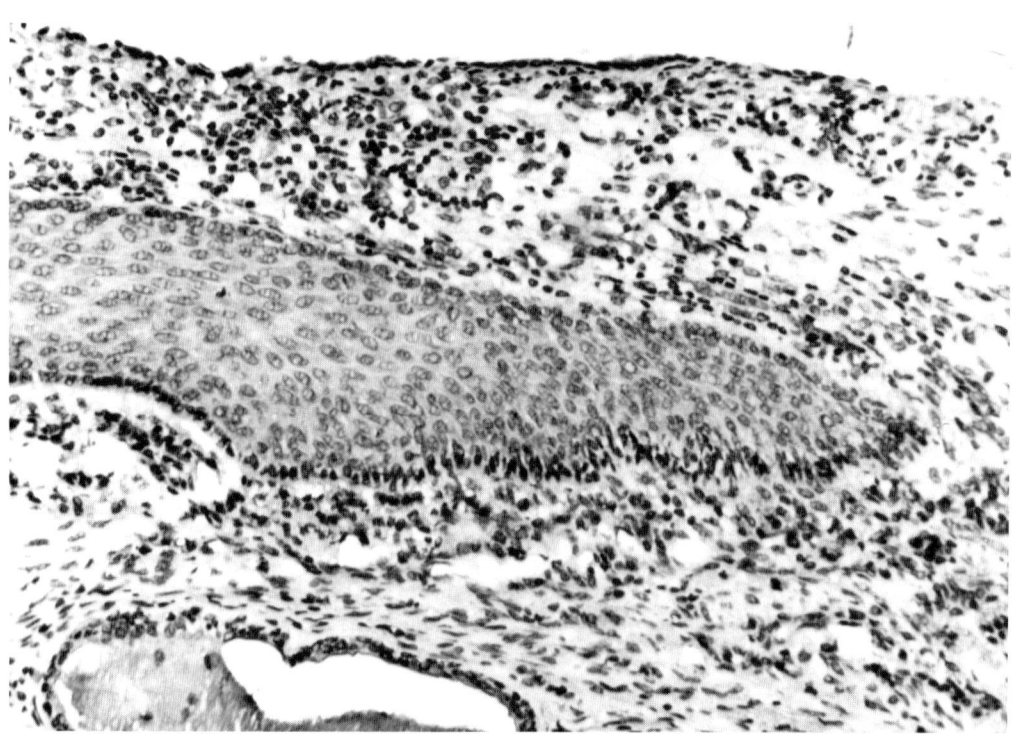

Figure 6.1. Example of unexpected finding of squamous epithelium in areas judged free of it during surgery. Papillary ingrowth of squamous epithelium into the stroma rich in inflammatory cells and covered by one-layer epithelium, in posterior part of tympanic cavity. *Bottom part* shows a large cyst. Hematoxylin-eosin stain, high magnification.

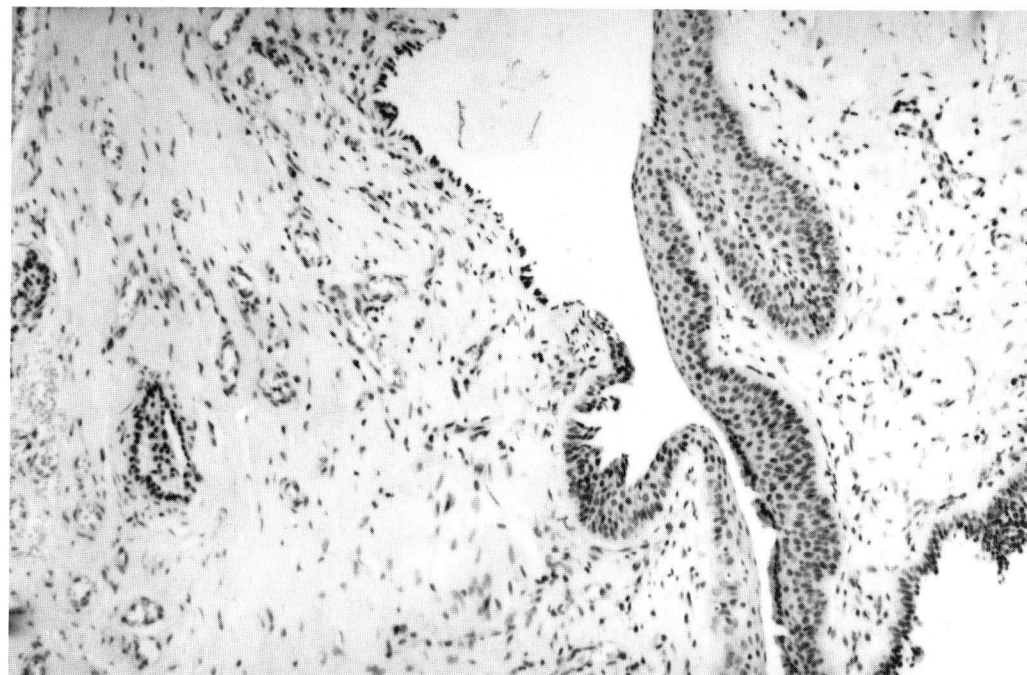

Figure 6.2. Example of unexpected finding of squamous epithelium in areas judged free of it during surgery. Migrating squamous epithelium joining smoothly with respiratory epithelium, in the anterior part of tympanic cavity, quite separate from the cholesteatoma proper. Hematoxylin-eosin stain, medium magnification.

There is other evidence to support this suggestion. One of my present associates (15) studied a series of 307 ears operated upon in the Helsinki clinic during the years 1964–1968. In this series, there were 183 ears in which an open, modified radical mastoidectomy without middle ear reconstruction was performed. After an average observation time of 9.4 years, the frequency of recurrent cholesteatoma was 6.4%. This figure was reached by very average surgeons and it is by far much better than the figures reported by the present day dedicated canal wall up ear surgeons. It is exactly of the same order that my dedicated canal wall down group has obtained employing tympanic and epitympanic reconstruction. This to me is the crucial point: even an average ear surgeon is safe if he elects to do a modified radical operation without reconstruction. A dedicated canal wall down surgeon is safe even if he reconstructs, because he has superior visibility to all areas of the operative fields and he can achieve total removal of mucosal squamous epithelium. Finally, canal wall up is worse because the surgeon's visibility to some areas is without question inferior, and both canal wall up and canal wall down surgeons are unsafe if they do not understand mucosal histopathology and routinely follow their own biopsies.

POSTOPERATIVE LATE HEARING RESULTS

Good postoperative hearing presupposes a functioning Eustachian tube. This is the primary prerequisite and all other reconstruction considerations are secondary as to final success. In comparing the results of various ear surgeons, much depends upon the case selection, what percentage of the ears had an intact pars tensa and only Sharpnell's membrane disease, as compared to the number of badly diseased tympanic clefts. The other consideration is the absence or presence of the stapes superstructure, combined with the previously mentioned two disease forms.

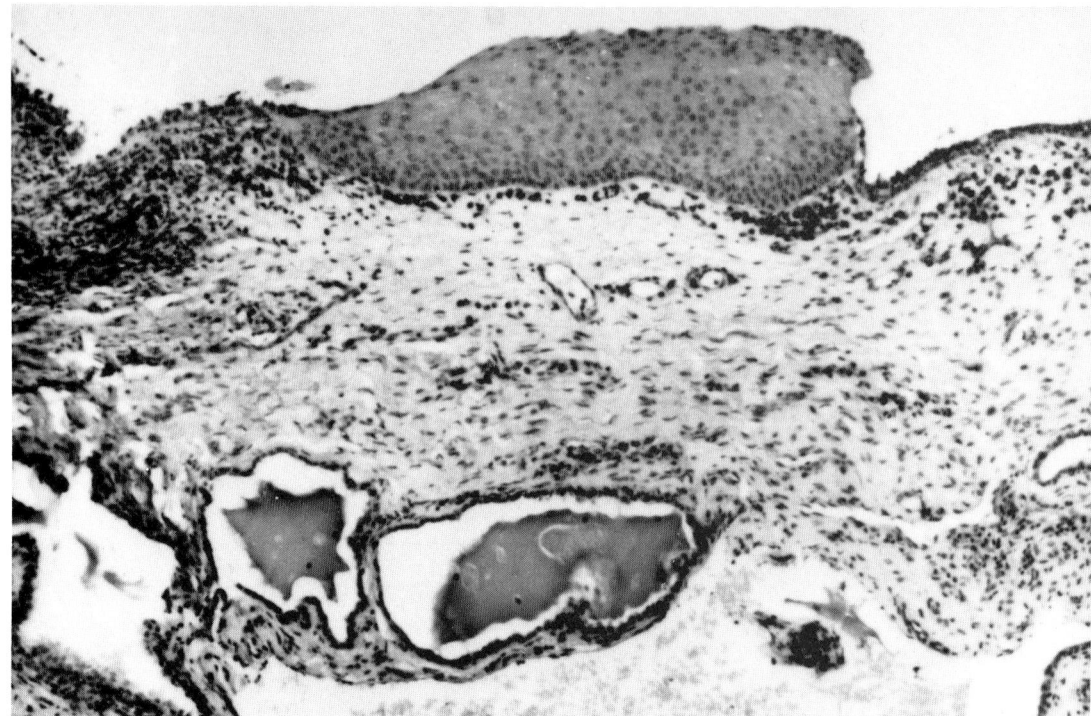

Figure 6.3. Example of unexpected finding of squamous epithelium in areas judged free of it during surgery. Islands of squamous epithelium, on facial nerve canal, surrounded by normal columnar epithelium on both sides. Inflammatory cell infiltration is seen on the *left*, large cysts at the *bottom*. Hematoxylin-eosin stain, low magnification.

All other variables have a minor influence upon the results.

In our early report (8) on the main material under discussion from the years 1964–1971, there are data that are in full agreement with the previous statements (Table 6.1). Table 6.1 shows only results with ossicular reconstruction (not those with foreign material) as this corresponds with present day methods. It is seen that all figures (average of 3 years' follow-up) show a definite improvement with the increasing tympanic pathology but in a diminishing degree.

The late figures reported by Ojala (9) for the whole series showed that in 8.8 years after surgery, there was an average further deterioration of hearing levels of about 6 dB. All groups, excepting that with no reconstruction, were still better than the preoperative average levels.

Another interesting finding must be pointed out from the series of Palmgren (15) with the 9.4 years of average observation time of cases of modified radical operation with open cavity. These results are shown in Table 6.2. Without reconstruction, there is an average further loss of 8.4 dB from the preoperative average level of 47.8 dB. In the subgroups, the figures were best in 36 years in which nature healed the perforation (41.2 dB) and worst in the 27 ears (66.6 dB) in which the middle ear was totally adhesive. However, in all subgroups, the postoperative results were worse than the preoperative figures.

These results of our various series followed for a long time testify that ossicular and middle ear reconstruction should be the aim of the surgeon because that is the only way to obtain hearing gain from the preoperative figures. However, this is also one of the dangers of chronic ear surgery because during reconstruction closes the

Table 6.1
Ossicular Reconstruction, 3-Year Follow-Up

	N	Preoperative	Postoperative
Incus transposition			
Mucosa preserved	121	41.7 dB	30.1 dB
Mucosa removed	59	51.3 dB	40.7 dB
Incus on footplate			
Mucosa preserved	23	48.3 dB	31.6 dB
Mucosa removed	20	56.5 dB	44.4 dB

Table 6.2
Hearing After Surgery Without Reconstruction

Operation type	Preoperative	Late
Modified radical (104 ears)	47.8 dB	56.2 dB
Nature healed perforation (36 ears)	37.4 dB	41.2 dB
Totally adhesive (27 ears)	53.4 dB	66.6 dB
Tympanomastoidectomy (74 ears)	46.4 dB	52.0 dB

middle ear and the attic. Microscopic evidence of the advancing front of the keratinizing squamous epithelium distant from the clinical cholesteatoma may not be familiar to the surgeon and he may elect to leave mucosa that does not look cholesteatomatous but nevertheless contains squamous epithelium. The out-of-the-ear migration of the surface keratin is no longer possible on closed ears and the result is a recurring cholesteatoma. To claim here, e.g., that the modified radical surgery procedure with obliteration is not safer than the canal wall up procedure in my opinion is misleading and shows the lack of knowledge of the behavior of the middle ear epithelial migration.

A final word about a second look. I cannot understand the feasibility of this routine procedure when the recurrent cholesteatoma in 12 years' evaluation with the exposure given by the modified radical mastoidectomy is around 6%. I think that surgeons with high recurrence figures should start anew with the modified radical operation, refresh their knowledge thoroughly in middle ear histopathology, and apply that knowledge in their everyday ear surgery. One cannot be a first class ear surgeon without being a pathologist at the same time.

References

1. Myers, D., and Schlosser, W.D. Anterior-posterior technique for treatment of chronic otitis media and mastoiditis. Laryngoscope 70: 78-83, 1960.
2. Jansen, C. The combined approach for tympanoplasty. J Laryngol Otol 82 779-793, 1968.
3. Guilford, F. R. Obliteration of the cavity and reconstruction of the auditory canal in temporal bone surgery. Trans Am Acad Ophthalmol Otolaryngol 65: 114-122, 1961.
4. Palva, T. Reconstruction of ear canal in surgery for chronic ear. Arch Otolaryngol 75: 329-334, 1962.
5. Palva, T. Surgery of chronic ear without cavity. Arch Otolaryngol 77: 570-580, 1963.
6. Palva, T., Palva, A., and Karja, J. Results with 2- or 3-legged wire columellization in chronic ear surgery. Ann Otol Rhinol Laryngol 80: 760-765, 1971.
7. Palva, T. Operative technique in mastoid obliteration. Acta Otolaryngol (Stockh) 75: 289-290, 1973.
8. Palva, T., Palva, A., and Kärjä, J. Ossicular reconstruction in chronic ear surgery. Arch Otolaryngol 98: 340-348, 1973.
9. Ojala, K. Late results of obliteration operation in chronic otitis media. Acta Universitatis Ouluensis, Ser. D. Medica No. 47; Ophthalmolgica et Oto-Rhino-Laryngologica 5: 1-106, 1979.

10. Palva, T., Palva, A., and Kärjä, J. Cavity obliteration and ear canal size. *Arch Otolaryngol* 92: 366–371, 1970.
11. Palva, T., and Mäkinen, J. The meatally based musculoperiosteal flap in cavity obliteration. *Arch Otolaryngol* 105: 377–380, 1979.
12. Palva, T. How I do it. An alternate use of TORP and PORP. *Laryngoscope* (In press).
13. Smyth, G.D.L. *Chronic Ear Disease.* Churchill Livingstone, New York, 1980. (Monographs in *Clin Otolaryngol* Vol. 2).
14. Palva, T., Palva, A., and Dammert, K. Middle ear mucosa and chronic ear disease. *Arch Otolaryngol* 87: 21–29, 1968.
15. Palmgren, O. Operationsresultat vid aktiv kronisk mellanöroninflammation. En klinisk studie vid lång observationstid. M.D. Thesis, University of Helsinki, p. 79, 1977.

CHAPTER 7

Total Reconstruction of the Ossicular Chain[1]

Ugo P. Fisch, M.D.

The goals of tympanoplasty are:
1. elimination of disease,
2. restoration of the Eustachian tube function,
3. reconstruction of the sound transformer mechanism of the middle ear.

The follow-up study of patients operated upon in the past 5 years for noncholesteatomatous chronic ear disease indicate that when the malleus, incus, and stapes arch are missing, the following factors contribute to improving the postoperative hearing results: epitympanectomy, preserved septal cartilage for reconstruction of the medial attic wall and reinforcement of the drum, thick silastic sheeting, transmastoid drainage, staging, and the use of TORP's. The majority of the mentioned measures aim at restoring aeration of the reconstructed tympanic cavity indicating that this still is the major problem when there is extensive destruction of ossicular tissue (1). Let us review the rationale for each one of the previously listed measures.

EPITYMPANECTOMY

Epitmypanectomy consists of removal of the malleus head, incus body, and tensor chorda fold as well as the exenteration of the supralabyrinthine cell tract. The aim of the procedure is to establish a wide communication between the anterior attic and the protympanum, thus reestablishing the superior ventilation route of the middle ear cleft (Fig. 7.1). B. Proctor (2) has demonstrated that the anterior attic space develops as a separate compartment which is limited by the superior malleolar fold, the malleus head, and the chorda tensor fold. A study carried out in our department on 30 normal human temporal bones has shown that the anterior attic space of the adult man is ventilated through an opening of the tensor chorda fold in only one-third of the cases (Fig. 7.2). In the remaining two-thirds of the cases, the chorda tensor fold is a closed membrane and the ventilation of the anterior attic takes place from the tympanic isthmus through a dehiscence of the superior malleolar fold. This situation explains why the aeration of the anterior attic may become critical in presence of middle ear infection. The accumulation of chronic, irreversible mucosal disease in the anterior attic (Fig. 7.3) can only be prevented by systematic epitympanectomy.

PRESERVED CARTILAGE FOR RECONSTRUCTION OF THE MEDIAL ATTIC WALL AND REINFORCEMENT OF THE DRUM

The superior and posterior canal wall is usually eroded at the tympanic rim in presence of extensive destruction of ossicular tissues. Septal cartilage preserved in a 1:5000 solution of cialit[2] is cut with a knife (no. 15 blade) in slices of 0.2–0.4 mm thickness. These are used to reconstruct the bony defect and reinforce the posterosuperior quadrant of the new tympanic membrane. Preserved septal cartilage

[1] The statistical analysis of the results has been carried out at the Biomedical Statistical Institute of the University of Zurich (according to the Wilcoxon test by Dr. H. Helfenstein).

[2] Composition:2-(aethyl-mercuri-mercapto)-benzoxazol-5-carbonacid sodium (ASID Bonz & Sohn GmbH, 8044 Unterschleissheim/W. Germany).

slides more easily between tissues and fresh tragal cartilage. Furthermore, it does incorporate into the skin and the tympanic membrane rather than fix to the underlying bone. A thick silastic sheeting placed in the middle ear helps keeping the sliced septal cartilage in position (Fig. 7.4).

TRANSMASTOID DRAINAGE

A 5 mm outer diameter polyethylene tubing that has been permamently bent in an angle of 110° by placing it over a curved metal stylus in an oven at 80°C is introduced into the antrum through a separate retroauricular incision (Fig. 7.5). The transmastoid drainage is helpful in removing wound secretion and providing ventilation of the middle ear in the immediate postoperative period. A suction tube of smaller diameter than that of the drain is used daily after surgery to remove fluid accumulating in the antrum. The drain is removed when fluid production has ceased

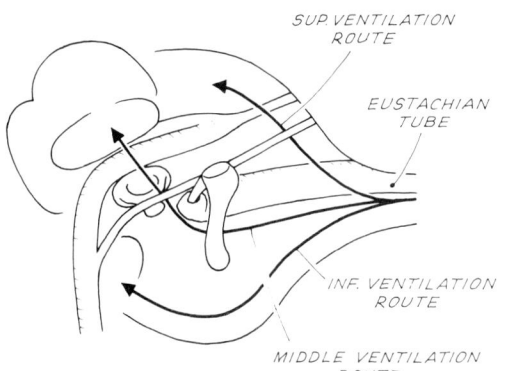

Figure 7.1. Ventilation routes to the middle ear cleft.

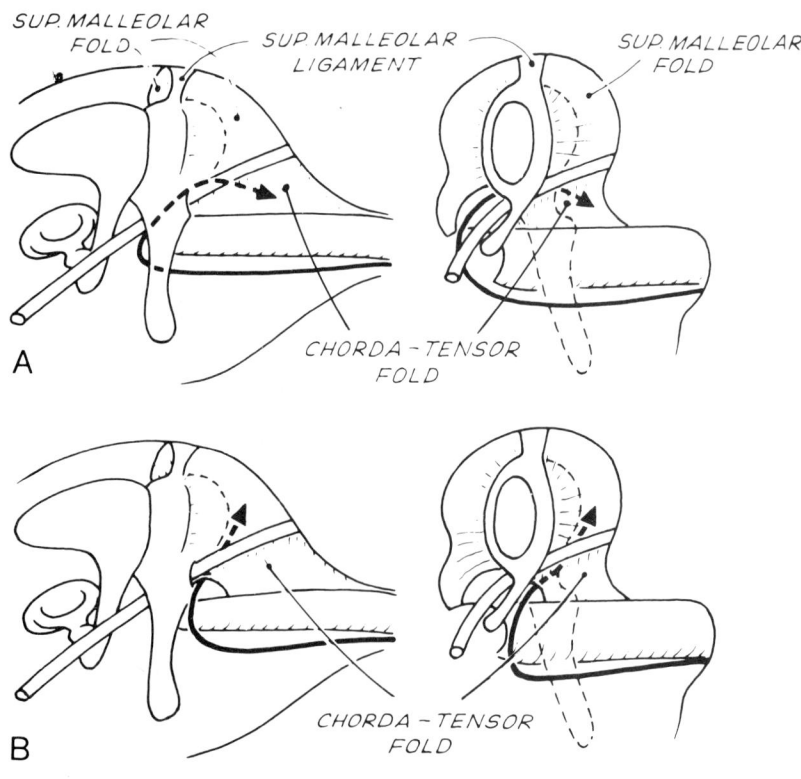

Figure 7.2. Results of the investigation carried out on 30 normal human temporal bones. A. The chorda tensor fold is closed in two-thirds of the cases. The ventilation of the anterior attic has to takeplace through a dehiscence of the superior malleolar fold, anteriorly to the tensor tympani tendon. B. The chorda tensor fold is open in one-third of the cases, assuring a direct ventilation of the anterior attic.

Total Reconstruction of Ossicular Chain 47

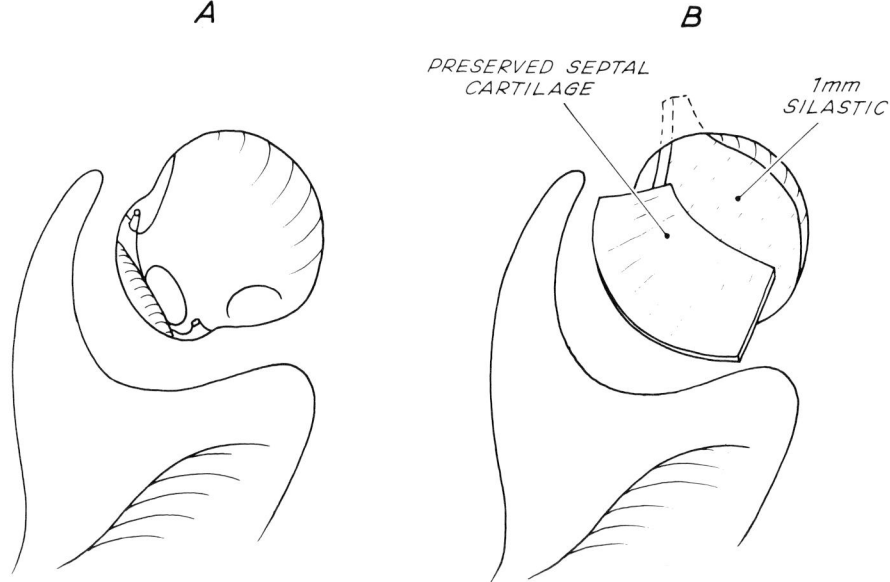

Figure 7.3. Reconstruction of the atrophic medial wall of the attic as well as of the posterosuperior quadrant of the drum with preserved septal cartilage.

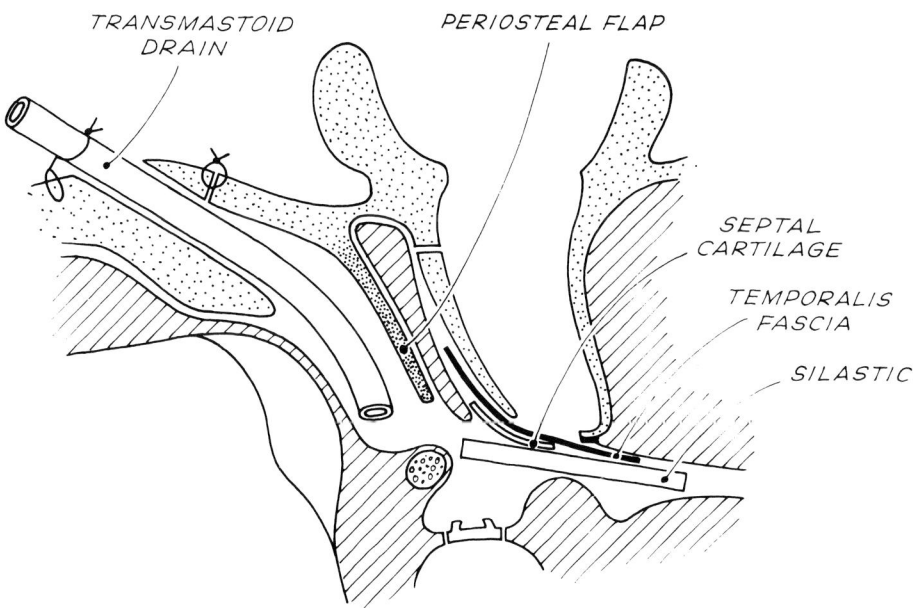

Figure 7.4. Position of the transmastoid drain at completion of surgery. Note that the silastic sheeting in the middle ear is supporting the septal cartilage and temporalis fascia.

and the Valsalva manoeuvre becomes positive (usually 4–8 days postoperatively).

The systematic use of epitympanectomy, the reconstruction of the posterosuperior tympanic rim and drum with septal cartilage as well as the transmastoid drainage have significantly reduced the number of posterosuperior or attic retractions ob-

48 Clinical Otology

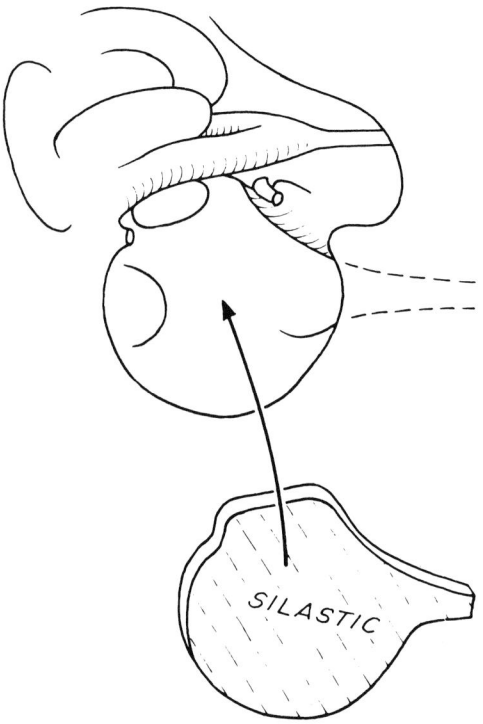

Figure 7.5. When the ossicular tissue is missing, the thick silastic sheeting is fashioned to fit into the entire middle ear cavity extending into the tympanic ostium of the Eustachian tube.

served at the 3 years' follow-up in 126 patients who underwent tympanomastoidectomy in presence of extensive destruction of the ossicular chain (Table 7.1).

STAGING

Sheehy and Crabtree (3) proposed that tympanoplasty should be performed as a planned two-stage procedure to obtain better hearing. This has also been our experience particularly when there was need for a total ossicular reconstruction. Al-

Table 7.1
Retraction Pockets Following Intact Canal Wall Technique (3 Years' Follow-Up, N = 126)[a]

Type of Surgery	Posterosuperior or Attic Retraction	
Malleus head in place	18/75	24%
Systematic epitympanectomy	4/51	8%[b]

[a] Patients underwent tympanomastoidectomy in presence of noncholesteatomous extensive destruction of the ossicular chain.
[b] $P = < 0.025$.

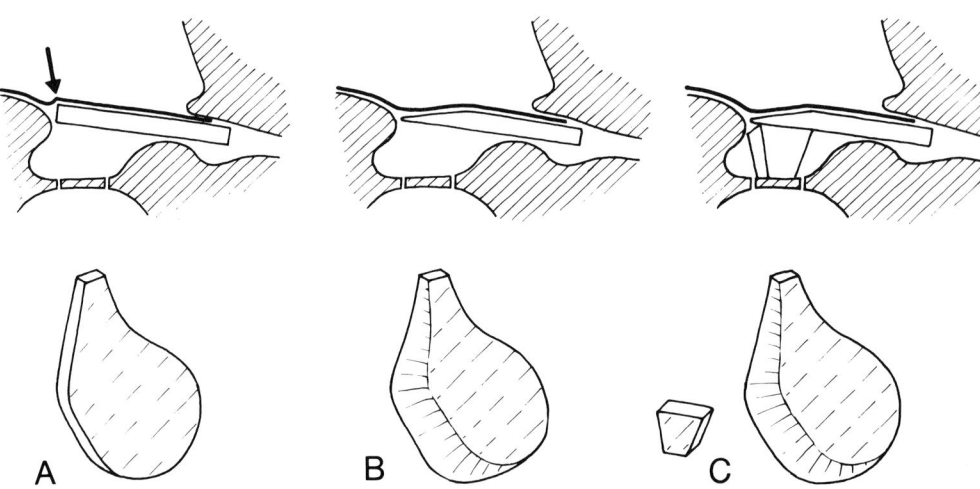

Figure 7.6. Sharp edges (A) of the silastic sheet must be avoided because of possible perforation of the drum. The excess of material is removed with curved tympanoplasty scissors (B). A small piece of silastic can be interposed between the stapes footplate and the larger middle ear silastic sheeting. This improves sound transmission while waiting for second stage surgery.

though still controversial (4), staging offers the undeniable advantage to permit evaluation of Eustachian tube function 6-12 months postoperatively and, therefore, to select good and reject bad candidates for ossicular reconstruction. Our criteria for staging (extensive destruction of middle ear mucosa, absence of malleus handle, stapes fixation with tympanic perforation, and residual cholesteatoma in middle ear or mastoid cavity) are similar to those proposed by Sheehy and Crabtree (3). In fact, we do stage every operation requiring total reconstruction of the ossicular chain when the tympanic membrane is not intact.

SILASTIC SHEETING

The use of thick plastic sheeting to improve reepithelization and avoid fibrosis in the middle ear cavity has also been advocated by Sheehy and Crabtree (3). In our series of patients, the use of 1 mm thick silastic sheeting has proven most beneficial. In contrary to the thin silastic that curled and wandered around depending on the caprice of scarring, thick silastic sheets remain in their original position if they are cut to fit exactly in the meso- and hypotympanum and to extend with a prolongation towards the tympanic ostium of the Eustachian tube (Fig. 7.6). Extension of the silastic sheeting into the mastoid cavity (3) is not necessary since reepithelization limited to the middle ear cavity is a more realistic and sufficient goal. Furthermore, silastic sheetings limited to the middle ear are easier to remove than those extending into the mastoid at second stage surgery. In order to avoid perforations of the tympanic membrane, sharp edges of the silastic must be removed with scissors (Fig. 7.7). The interposition of a small piece of silastic over the mobile footplate may improve the hearing while waiting for second stage surgery.

Alternate cuts may be used to break the rigidity of the silastic sheeting when the axis of the Eustachian tube is not in the same plane as the mesotympanum (Fig. 7.8).

USE OF TORP's

Table 7.2 shows that TORP's have significantly increased the number of patients with an airbone gap of 20 dB or less at the 1 year's follow-up in comparison to

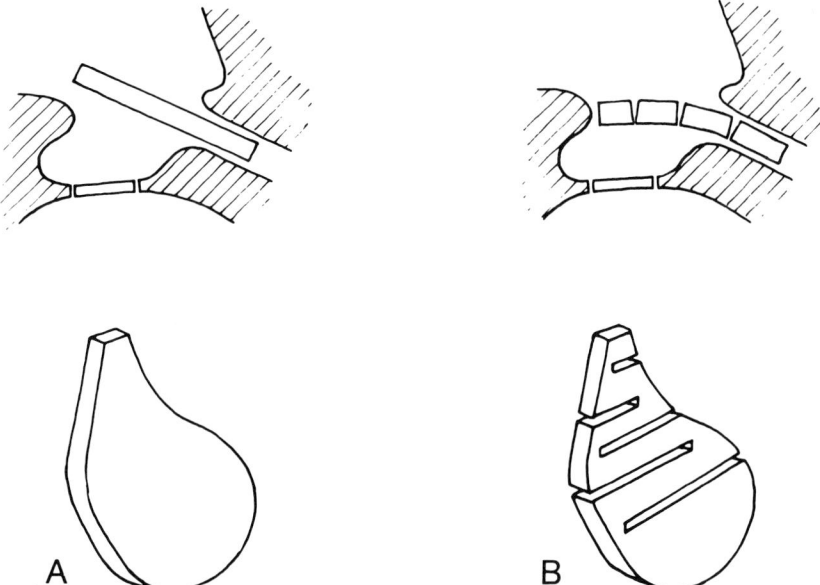

Figure 7.7. When the axis of the Eustachian tube does not allow proper fitting of the silastic sheeting into the middle ear cavity (*A*), alternate cuts (*B*) are used to reduce its rigidity.

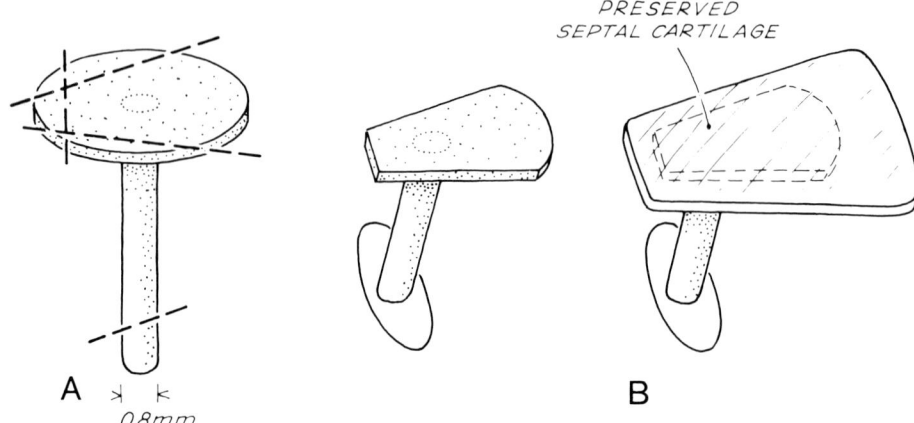

Figure 7.8. Transformation of the columella type TORP in a L-form. The lever action of the L-TORP is increased by adding preserved septal cartilage (B). The inclination of the prosthesis over the footplate is determined by the plane in which the shaft is cut to the desired length (A).

Table 7.2
Results of Total Ossicular Reconstruction (1 Year's Follow-Up)[a]

Postoperative Air-Bone Gap (dB)	Homologous Ossicles (N = 92)	TORP (N = 102)	P
0–10	4%	11%	
	17%	50%	<0.001
0–20	13%	39%	
0–30	46%	56%	NS
>30	54%	44%	NS

[a] TORP's have significantly increased the number of patients with an air-bone gap of 20 dB or less at the 1 year follow-up in comparison to homologous ossicles.

homologous ossicles. The advantage of the plastipore TORP is its nonrigid, porous structure.

The plasticity of the TORP can be increased by transforming the columella type in a "L-form" (Fig. 7.8). The lever action of the L-shaped head of the TORP may be increased by adding a piece of preserved septal cartilage that also prevents extrusion. The inclination of the prosthesis over the footplate is determined by the plane in which the shaft is cut to the desired length. The ideal diameter of the TORP's shaft has been found to be 0.8 mm (1 mm being too thick and 0.6 mm too thin). The modified L-TORP's have been used in the footplate to drum and in the vestibulum to drum situations. In the latter case, sealing off the oval window was obtained with pressed perichondrium. The same material was also used over the mobile footplate to improve the attachment between TORP shaft and the stapes footplate. At present, we investigate whether biocompatible fibrinogen glue[3] is helpful in stabilizing the TORP following reconstruction.

The 1 year's follow-up results in 56 patients with the footplate to drum reconstructions are shown in Table 7.3. At 1 year, there is a significantly higher number of patients with a postoperative airbone gap of 0–10 dB in the wall up versus the wall down situation. In the vestibulum to drum situation (Table 7.4), the 1 year's follow-up study also shows a significantly higher number of 0–30 dB airbone gap closures when the canal wall is left up rather than taken down.

[3] Immuno A.G., Börsenstr. 14,8001 Zurich/Switzerland.

Table 7.3
Results of TORP's in Total Ossicular Reconstruction (Footplate to Drum, N = 56)

Postoperative Air-Bone Gap (dB)	Wall Up	Wall Down	P
0–10	(7/37) 19%	(0/19) 0%	<0.05
0–20	(20/37) 54%	(7/19) 37%	NS
0–30	(28/37) 76%	(10/19) 53%	NS
>30	(9/37) 24%	(0/19) 47%	NS

Table 7.4
Results of TORP's in Total Ossicular Reconstruction (Vestibulum to Drum, N = 26)

Postoperative Air-Bone Gap (dB)	Wall Up	Wall Down	P
0–10	(3/19) 16%	(0/7) 0%	NS
0–20	(7/19) 37%	(1/7) 14%	NS
0–30	(11/19) 58%	(1/7) 14%	<0.05
>30	(8/19) 42%	(6/7) 86%	<0.05

Altogether, the hearing results were better when the footplate was left in situ than following stapedectomy (Tables 7.3 and 7.4).

CONCLUSIONS

1. Systematic epitympanectomy, preserved cartilage to reconstruct the posterosuperior tympanic rim and quadrant of the drum, thick silastic sheeting, and transmastoid drainage have significantly reduced the number of postoperative drum restrictions when there was extensive destruction of ossicular tissue.

2. Staging with thick silastic sheeting and 0.8 mm TORP's have significantly improved the functional results of total reconstruction of the ossicular chain in comparison to homologous ossicles.

3. The functional results of staged reconstruction with L-TORP's are significantly better when the canal wall is left up rather than taken down.

4. In spite of the mentioned progresses, total reconstruction of the ossicular chain is still far from being satisfactory and needs further improvement.

References

1. Fisch, U. *Tympanoplasty and Stapedectomy, A Manual of Techniques.* Thieme-Stratton Inc., New York, 1980.
2. Proctor, B. The development of the middle ear spaces and their surgical significance. *J Laryngol* 78: 631–648, 1964.
3. Sheehy, J.L., and Crabtree, J.A. Tympanoplasty, staging the operation. *Laryngoscope* 83: 1594–1621, 1973.
4. Smyth, G.D.L. *Chronic Ear Disease.* Churchill, Livingstone, New York, 1980.

CHAPTER 8
Prefabricated Allograft Ossiculoplasty
Victor Goodhill, M.D., F.A.C.S.

Correction of ossicular defects is indicated in congenital, traumatic, and post-infection lesions. The most common lesion requiring ossiculoplasty is an absent or necrotic incus. If there is a mobile tympanic membrane, malleus and stapes, or stapes footplate, ossiculoplastic reconstruction is possible. This can be accomplished in a number of ways, including use of 1. resculptured incus autograft (Fig. 8.1); 2. tragal cartilage autograft; 3. prefabricated preserved allograft ossicle; and 4. commercially available metal, plastic, or ceramic prostheses. Tympanoplasty frequently is required either simultaneously or as a separate procedure.

Tragal cartilage has a limited application in ossiculoplasty, because of its lesser stiffness, but it has a place in our armamentarium. It can be used especially in Type III tympanoplasty in shallow tympanum conditions, as a short cartilage columella (Fig. 8.2) with or without attached perichondrium. Its lateral end may be in contact with tympanic membrane umbo, or with a perichondrial or fascia graft tympanic membrane replacement.

Where there is no tympanic membrane,

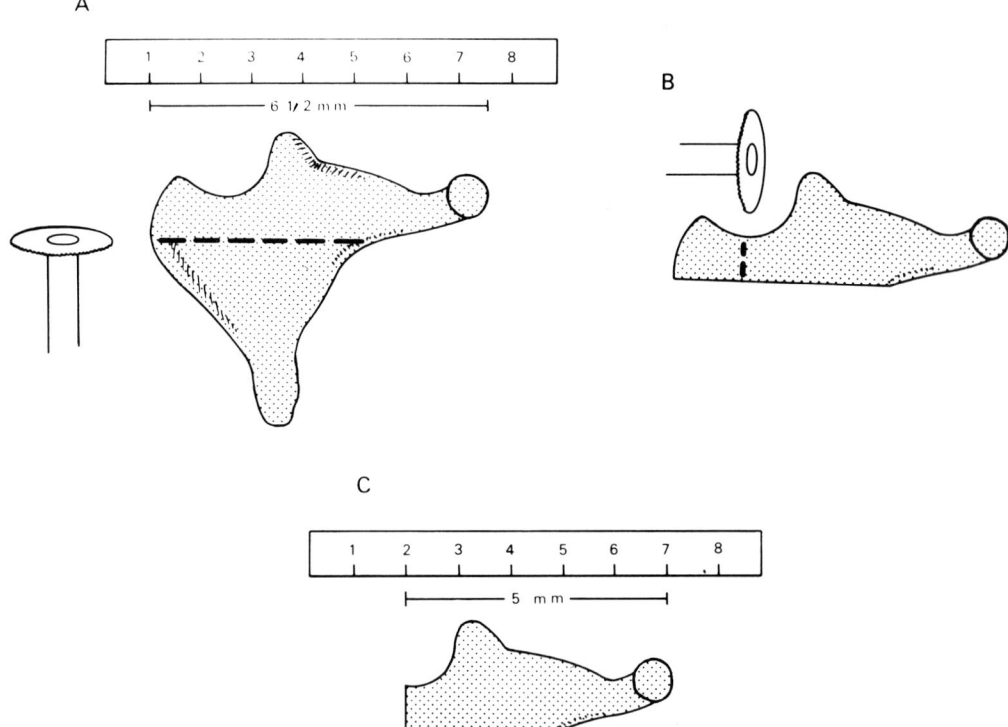

Figure 8.1. Autogenous incus remodeling for use in ossiculoplasty.

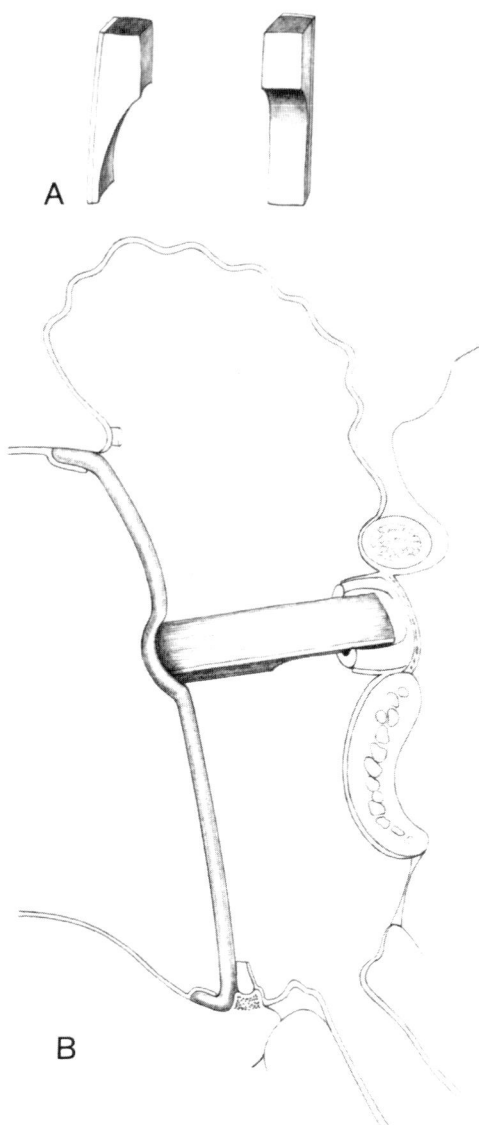

Figure 8.2. *A.* Prepared cartilage columella with perichondrial surface still intact on one side. *B.* Conventional cartilage columella in position on stapedial footplate, its lateral extremity in contact with convexity of perichondrial autograft. (Reproduced from Goodhill, V. *Arch Otolaryngol*).

a composite T-cartilage perichondrial graft is prepared by perichondrial elevation from both surfaces of a large tragal graft with tailoring and shaping preoperatively of a T-graft still attached to its own perichondrium. (Fig. 8.3)

Allograft (homograft) preserved ossicles have been used widely in recent years. Prefabricated allograft ossicular columellae have been made in our temporal bone laboratory. We define the columella as the interposed structure between the malleus and either the stapedial capitulum or the footplate. A "short" columella is interposed between malleus and stapedial capitulum. A "long" columella is interposed between the malleus and footplate or neofootplate membrane.

The short or long ossicular columella is "locked" into a surgically prepared malleal trough laterally (Fig. 8.4). A malleal neck trough, approximately 1 × 1.5 mm, is made with cutting and/or diamond burrs above the crossover region of the chorda tympani and malleus.

The short golf-tee columella is prefabricated from an allograft malleus. The long rod columella is prefabricated from an allograft incus. Both the long and the short columella may be prepared from either right or left ossicles for use on either side. (Fig. 8.5).

The prefabrication is carried out with the use of a large diamond burr. The ossicle may be hand held or held in a forceps. Since the essential process is that of sculpture, technical dexterity is obviously necessary.

SHORT COLUMELLA (GOLF-TEE)—MALLEAL TROUGH TO STAPES

A malleus allograft is used. The final shape is an elongated cone with the base (medial end) hollowed out to form a golf-tee shape to fit over the capitulum, neck, and stapes tendon. The dimensions vary from 3.5–4.5 mm in overall length. The golf-tee shape is approximately 1.50–1.75 mm in diameter. The lateral rod end for attachment to the malleal trough is 0.75 mm in diameter, and is scored to provide a slightly rough surface to expedite fibrous tissue anchorage.

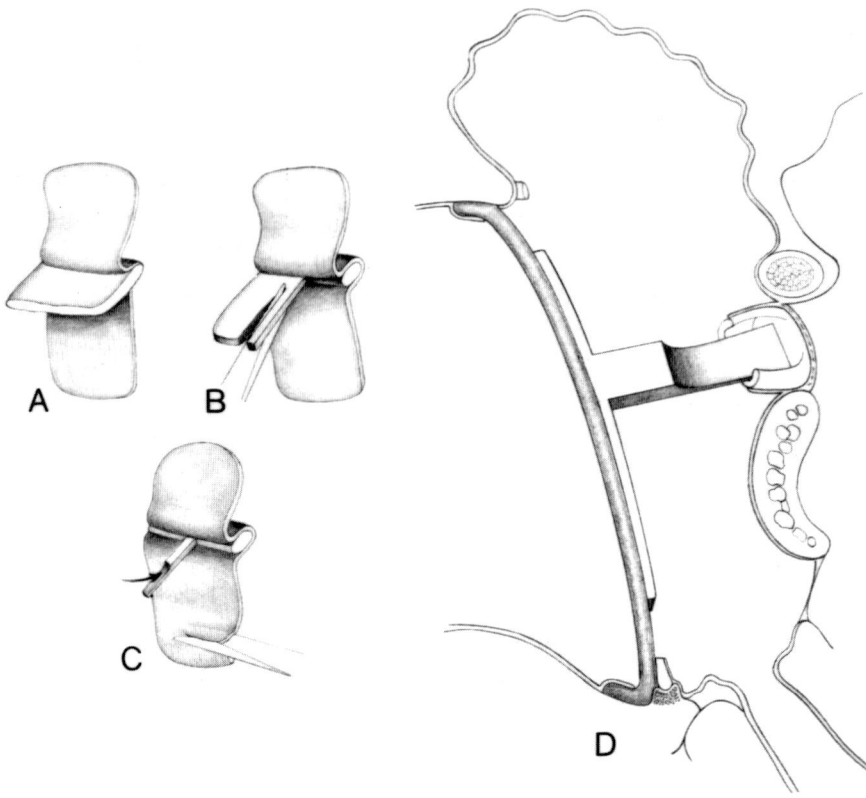

Figure 8.3. *A.* Perichondrium elevated from both surfaces of tragal cartilage. *B.* Tailoring of tragal cartilate to create T-cartilage perichondrial composite graft. *C.* Medial aspect of columella thinned and perichondrium shaped to proper size. *D.* T-cartilage perichondrial graft in place, its medial aspect in contact with mobile stapedial footplate after partial amputation of crura. Note adequate tympanic air space. (Reproduced from Goodhill, V. *Arch Otolaryngol*).

LONG COLUMELLA (ROD)—MALLEAL TROUGH TO OVAL WINDOW

An incus allograft is used. The final shape is that of a slightly tapered rod. The length of the rod varies from 5.75–6.5 mm. The lateral end is identical in measurement to that of the golf-tee, 0.75–1.0 mm in diameter. The medial end is slightly narrower, 0.65–0.8 mm.

BONE "RIVET" COLUMELLA

In relatively unusual instances to be described later, rivet modifications of both long and short columellae may be necessary if malleal trough preparation is not feasible. Lateral attachment is secured by deliberate penetration through the perimanubrial region of the pars tensa. This columella is capped with a scored head.

SURGICAL TECHNIQUES—INDICATIONS AND CONTRAINDICATIONS

The malleal trough technique is adaptable to most forms of repair problems, i.e., intact tympanic membrane or large or small tympanic membrane perforations in any location (either the pars tensa or the pars flaccida). It is assumed that adequate

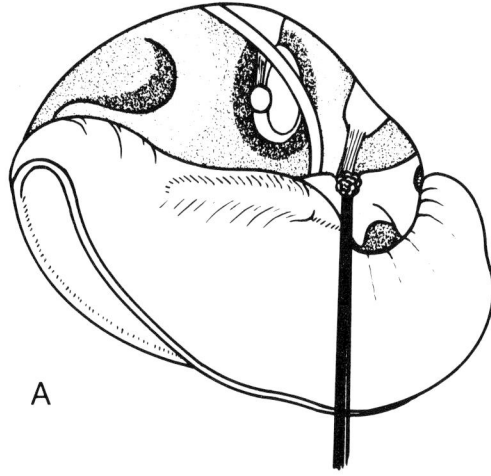

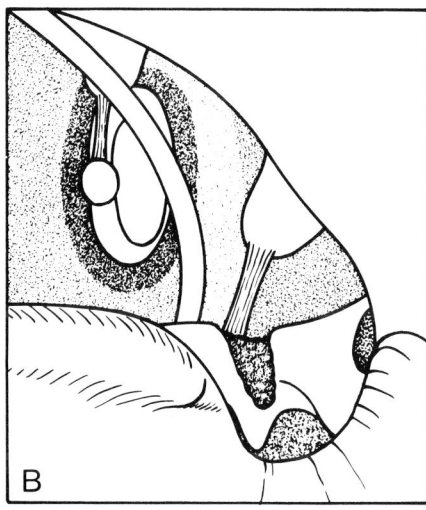

Figure 8.4. A. Beginning preparation of malleal trough, lateral to the level of insertion of tensor tympani tendon, and superior to chorda tympani malleal crossover. B. Completed trough in malleal neck and short process. (Reproduced from Goodhill, V. *Trans Am Acad Ophthal Otolaryngol* 78: ORL 411–422, 1974.)

removal of the lesion has preceded the reconstruction, either as a combined or as a staged procedure. The essential anatomic prerequisite is an intact mobile tympanic membrane, head, neck, and short process of the malleus, and an intact tensor tympani tendon. It is also desirable, for stabilization purposes, that the epitympanic pouch system (Prussak's pouch and the pouch of von Troltsch) and anterior ligament and tympanic folds be intact.

An appropriate columella is selected from the sterile collection available, after middle ear measurements have been obtained.

The malleal trough is prepared by elevating medial malleal periosteum. Soft tissues are reflected and a "trough" approximately 2.00 × 1.75 mm is created with cutting burrs. It is tailored in size and contoured to fit the selected allograft ossicle.

The lateral end of the short or long columella is fitted into the trough (Fig. 8.6 A and B) so that it engages snugly. Minor modifications of trough dimensions are made if necessary to secure snug engagement.

If there is an inadequacy in pars flaccida tissue components, the lateral end of the columella in the trough should be covered by a tragal cartilage-perichondrium graft (Fig. 8.6 C). The cartilage stopple will act as "cork" over the shaft in the trough. The perichondrium will protect the trough-columella area and, in turn is covered laterally by reflection of the remaining components of the posterior pars flaccida, the soft tissues of von Troltsch's and Prussak's spaces. If there is a posterior perforation, the shaft-trough-cartilage-perichondrium area is covered by a perichondrial graft used to repair the tympanic membrane defect.

When a short golf-tee columella is used, the concavity is manipulated into good contact with the stapes capitululm. With a long rod columella, the medial end is placed over the oval window. If the footplate is intact, gentle elevation of the mucoperiosteum should be followed by placement of two 1 × 1 mm perichondrial grafts on the footplate to stabilize the rod.

If there is a pre-existing fibrous oval window as a result of either surgical repair following removal of the bony footplate or spontaneous neomembrane regeneration of the oval window, the area must be sufficiently thick to receive the rod without danger of perforation. If it is thin, it should

56 Clinical Otology

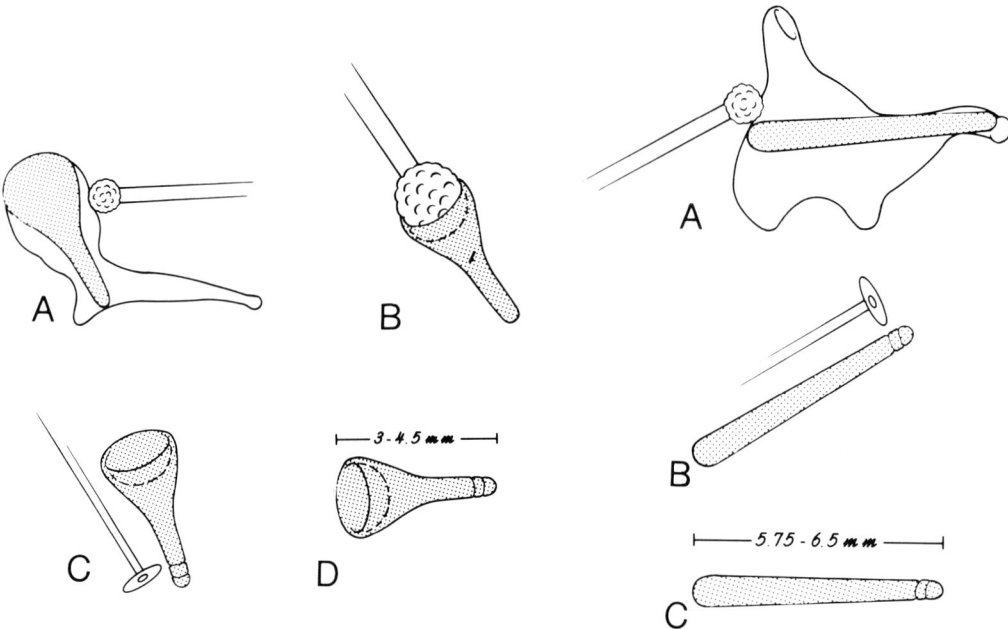

Figure 8.5. *Left side:* step by step preparation of golf-tee allograft from malleus. *Right side:* step-by-step preparation of rod allograft from incus. (Reproduced from Goodhill, V. R Soc Med).

be covered by a concave canoe-shaped fresh perichondrial graft.

Special Problems

The anatomic prerequisite for malleal trough columellae is an intact mobile head, neck, and short process of the malleus, and an intact tensor tympani tendon. If the manubrium has no attachment to these epitympanic structures, or if the malleal head is absent or separated from the neck and short process, the trough approach may not be possible.

One alternative is the rivet perimanubrial technique, which utilizes the principle of a projecting columella, the lateral end of which is exterior to the tympanic membrane. Following diamond burr dermabrasion of the perimanubrial area, a sharp stab incision, 2.5 mm in length, is made through the perimanubrial periosteum and radial fibers above the umbo.

In the long columella application (no stapes arch), the rod is introduced laterally through this stab. It is topped with a flat or scored "head" to maintain contact with the manubrium and to prevent it from slipping. Its medial end is placed as described before, either on a mobile footplate or oval window perichondrial graft (Fig. 8.7 A).

If the stapes if present, a short columella is introduced from a medial approach, the scored head or "cap" being introduced through the slit. The medial placement of the saddle on the stapes is as previously described (Fig. 8.7 B). The presenting cap lateral to the tympanic membrane, in either the long or the short columella, is covered by a small prichondrial graft (Fig. 8.7 C and D).

Another alternative is the use of a crutch-golf-tee or a crutch-rod prefabricated columella. The crutch portion is placed laterally, in continuity with mobile manubrium. Friction forces are used to maintain slight tension between the crutch-manubrium region and the footplate region.

Long range viability of ossicular allo-

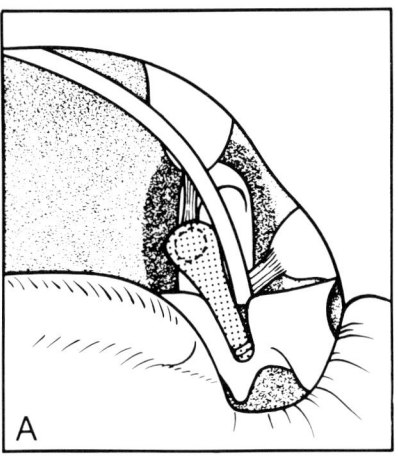
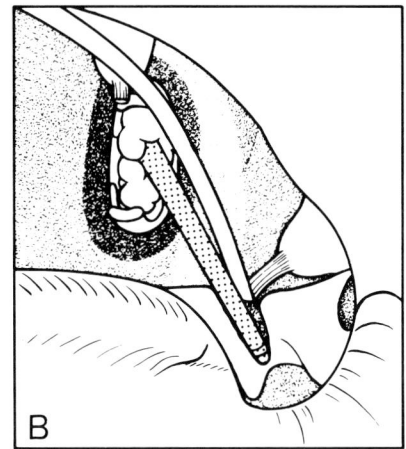
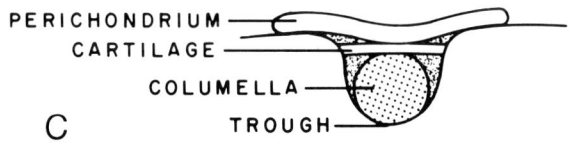

Figure 8.6. A. Golf-tee columella in position over stapedial capitulum. B. Rod columella in position on footplate surrounded by tissue grafts for stabilization. C. Cross section of trough columella junction showing closure of trough either by reflected soft tissue posterior flap or by use of cartilage perichondrium "stopple." (Reproduced from Goodhill, V. *Trans Am Acad Ophthal Otolaryngol* 78: ORL 411–422, 1974.)

grafts remains an unanswered question. I should like to present data on an interesting case.

Case History

R.L., a 77-year-old lady, had a persistent, chronic right otorrhea and episodic left otorrhea since childhood, with a severe bilateral mixed hearing loss; with right ear speech reception threshold (SRT) of 78 dB and SDS of 52%, and left ear SRT of 90 dB and SDS of 20%. A right mastoid tympanoplasty had been performed unsuccessfully elsewhere at age 62. There was a large suppurating right keratoma (cholesteatoma). There was a left scarred tympanosclerotic, but intact tympanic membrane. The draining right ear was her only potentially useful ear with a barely adequate speech discrimination score. However, hearing aids had been tried on a number of occasions without success.

Since she was an active lady in fairly good health except for occasional, well-controlled angina, who was unable to hear in either ear, a decision was made to explore the left ear which was the poorer ear but was dry. A left tympanotomy under local anesthesia was totally uneventful and she was discharged 24 hours postoperatively.

Operative findings included extensive tympanosclerosis involving the tympanic membrane. All three ossicles were fixed by panossicular fixation, with ossicular joints obliterated by tympanosclerosis. The lateral fixation was corrected by a drill-out, separating malleal head from manubrium. Incus was removed resulting in a mobile tympanic membrane and

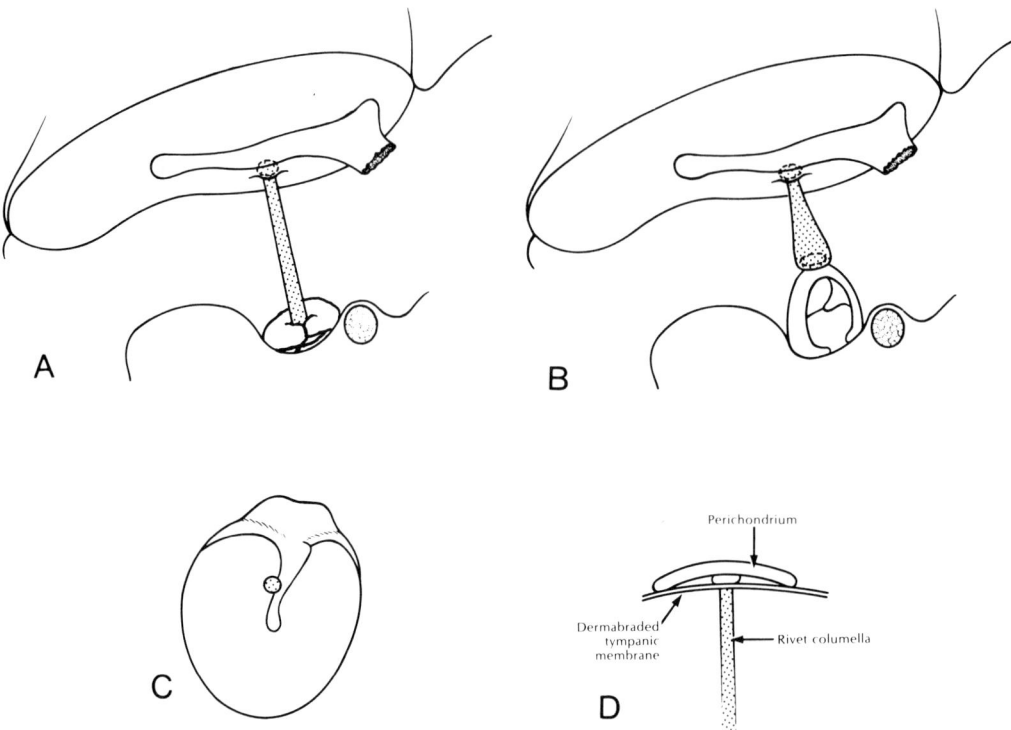

Figure 8.7. *A.* Rod columella inserted through perimanubrial slit in contact with footplate. *B.* Saddle columella inserted through perimanubrial slit in contact with stapedial capitulum. *C.* Otoscopic view of projecting cap rivet of either rod or saddle columella. *D.* Cross section of rivet columella showing cap projecting through perimanubrial slit in previously dermabraded tympanic membrane. Cap covered by small perichondrium graft on to dermabraded pars tensa. (Reproduced from Goodhill, V. *Trans Am Acad Ophthal Otalaryngol* 78: ORL 411–422, 1974.)

umbo. The fixed arch of the stapes and its footplate was removed and the oval window sealed with perichondrium. A prefabricated 6 mm rivet columella allograft was pushed (Fig 8.8) through a small perimanubrial slit in the dermabraded tympanic membrane and made contact medially with the oval window perichondrial graft. The lateral exposed part of the rivet (Fig. 8.9) was covered with a perichondrium graft held in place by a Gelfilm disc.

Postoperatively, there was a marked gain in hearing which stabilized at 34 dB with 68% SDS. Six months later, a small portion (1.5 mm long) of the allograft rod was seen protruding through the umbo region of the tympanic membrane. It was easily amputated with a cup forceps and removed, and sent to the Temporal Bone Laboratory for study. When examined several days later, the tympanic membrane was intact and the hearing remained unchanged.

Adequate unaided hearing was maintained until she died 17 months later. When seen 4 months before death, both ears were dry and the left hearing level was unchanged.

She died at the UCLA Hospital following a sudden acute angina and coronary thrombosis. The temporal bones were removed and sent to our laboratory.

A motion picture of this case was shown at the time of presentation of this paper at

Prefabricated Allograft Ossiculoplasty 59

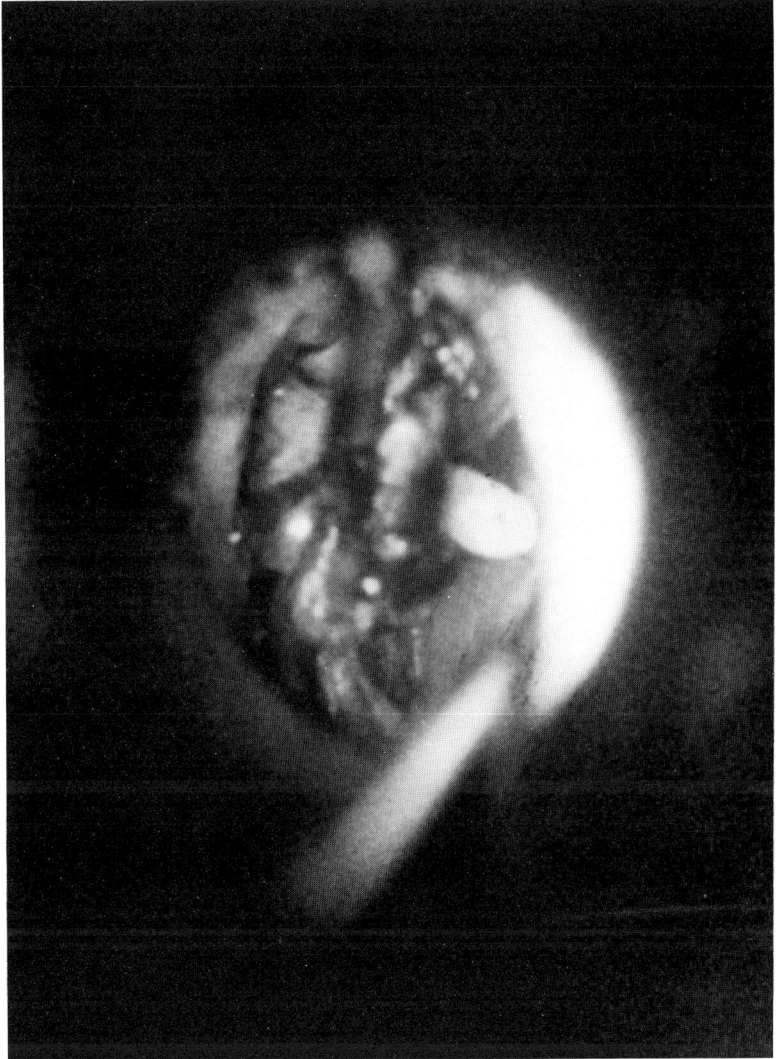

Figure 8.8. Prefabricated allograft ossiculoplasty, showing allograft pushed through tympanic membrane into middle ear.

the 1981 University of Minnesota Third Annual International Symposium on Clinical Otology. In this film, both operative findings and postmortem status were demonstrated.

When the temporal bone was received in our laboratory, I turned a classic tympanotomy flap after inspecting the tympanic membrane. The columella-tympanic membrane contact area was totally covered by intact epithelium. Within the tympanic cavity, the allograft columella, covered by mucosa, was found to be intact from the tympanic membrane to the oval window. This laboratory procedure was also demonstrated in the film.

The temporal bones were sectioned and studied in the UCLA Temporal Bone Laboratories by my colleague, Dr. Ruth Gussen.

In Figure 8.10, the oval window is sealed by irregularly-shaped collagenous tissue

60 Clinical Otology

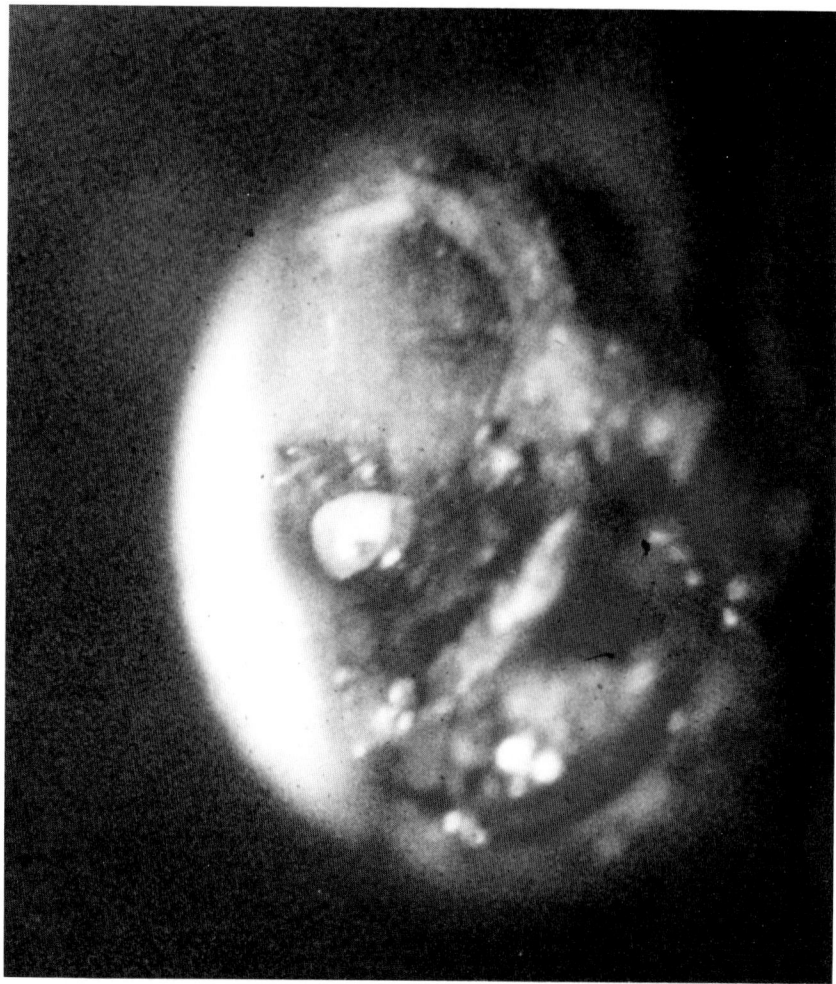

Figure 8.9. Prefabricated allograft ossiculoplasty showing lateral exposed rivet head.

which protrudes slightly into the vestibule and contains the superomedial portion of the bone allograft. From this section, a narrow fibrous band extends across the middle ear to the posterior portion of the tympanic membrane and in subsequent sections, will be seen to overlie the graft. Note tympanosclerotic involvement of the anterior and posterior oval window margins and of the mucosa overlying the facial nerve canal. The tympanic membrane is thickened by fibrous tissue.

In Figure 8.11, at a deeper level, but still in the oval window region, a portion of the bone allograft extends across the middle ear. Fibrous channels containing cells are present, extending into the bone from the surface.

In Figure 8.12, there is fibrous thickening on the posterior surface of the graft that will be seen later to be continuous with the stapedius tendon.

In Figure 8.13, the stapedius tendon is seen now attached to the graft.

In Figure 8.14, the tendon is near the posterior wall and this cut of the graft is also seen attached to the tympanic membrane by fibrous tissue.

In Figure 8.15, the bone allograft is seen embedded in the substance of the tym-

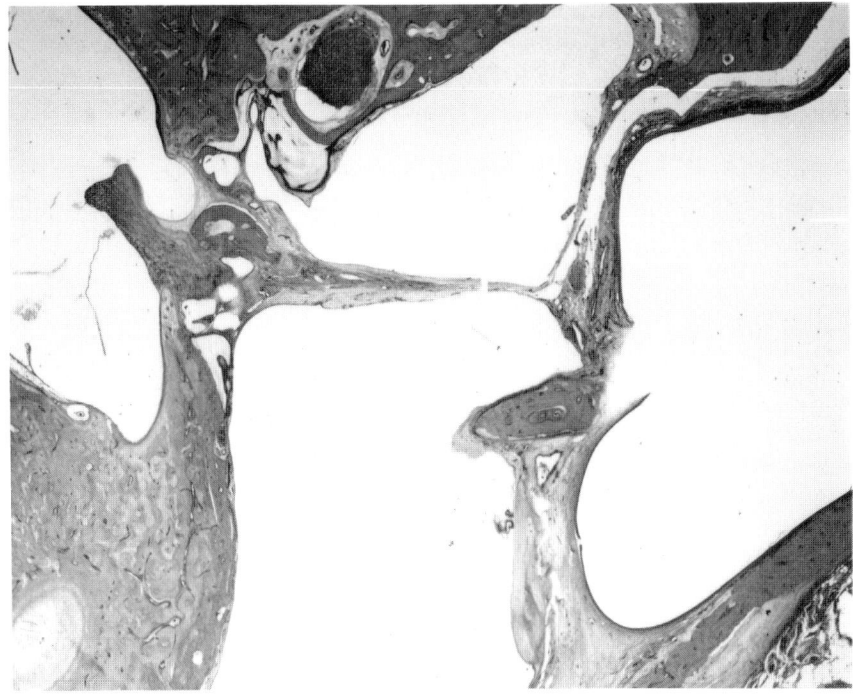

Figure 8.10. The oval window is sealed by irregularly shaped collagenous tissue which protrudes slightly into the vestibule and contains the superomedial portion of the bone allograft. From this section, a narrow fibrous band extends across the middle ear to the posterior portion of the tympanic membrane, and in subsequent sections will be seen to overlie the graft. Note tympanosclerotic involvement of the anterior and posterior oval window margins and of the mucosa overlying the facial nerve canal. The tympanic membrane is thickened by fibrous tissue.

panic membrane as it has been serially followed across the middle ear. The tympanic membrane is considerably thickened by fibrous tissue and by a tympanosclerotic plaque on its middle ear surface.

In Figure 8.16, in this high power view, the bone allograft is almost completely acellular, except near the surface, in some regions, where small numbers of lacunae contain cells. The vascular channels within the bone, however, contain cells and these areas are continuous with cellular, fibrous tissue on the graft surface.

In Figure 8.17, we see a normal incus section from a 78-year-old individual for comparison. One seems mostly empty lacunae, save for occasional perivascular regions where bone cells are present.

In Figure 8.18, we see a section of the postoperative exteriorized fragment of bone allograft which is completely nonviable. No bone cells are evident. Small amounts of cellular fibrous tissue extend into the graft near the surface.

DISCUSSION

This essentially inert and devitalized allograft bone rod functioned well for 17 months.

Otologic surgeons who have been using ossicular allografts with good hearing results and unextruded ossicles cannot predict long-range survival of such nonvital bone grafts. The vast majority of allografts used by me and my colleagues are articu-

62 Clinical Otology

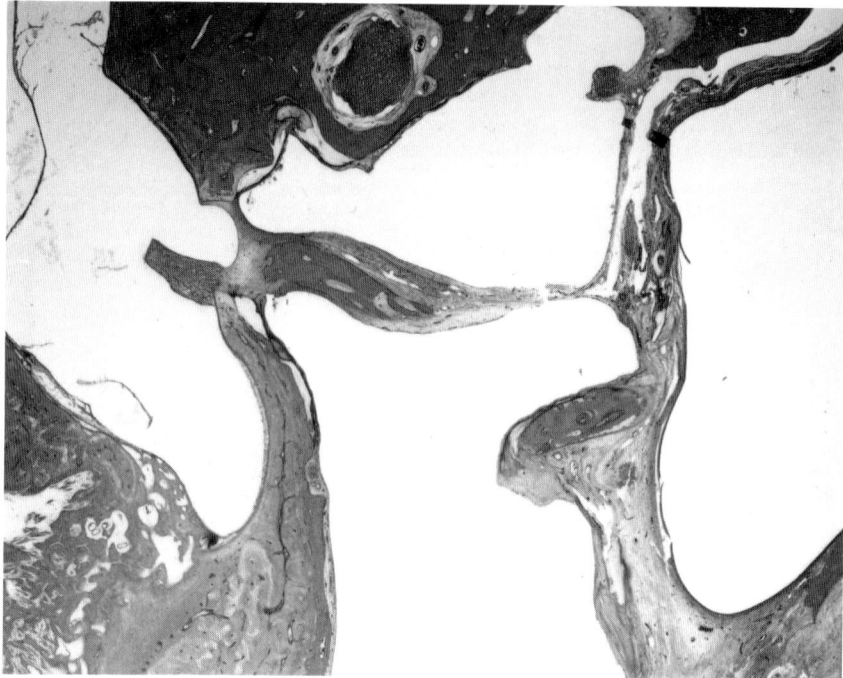

Figure 8.11. At a deeper level, but still in the oval window region, a portion of the bone allograft extends across the middle ear. Fibrous channels containing cells are present, extending into the bone from the surface.

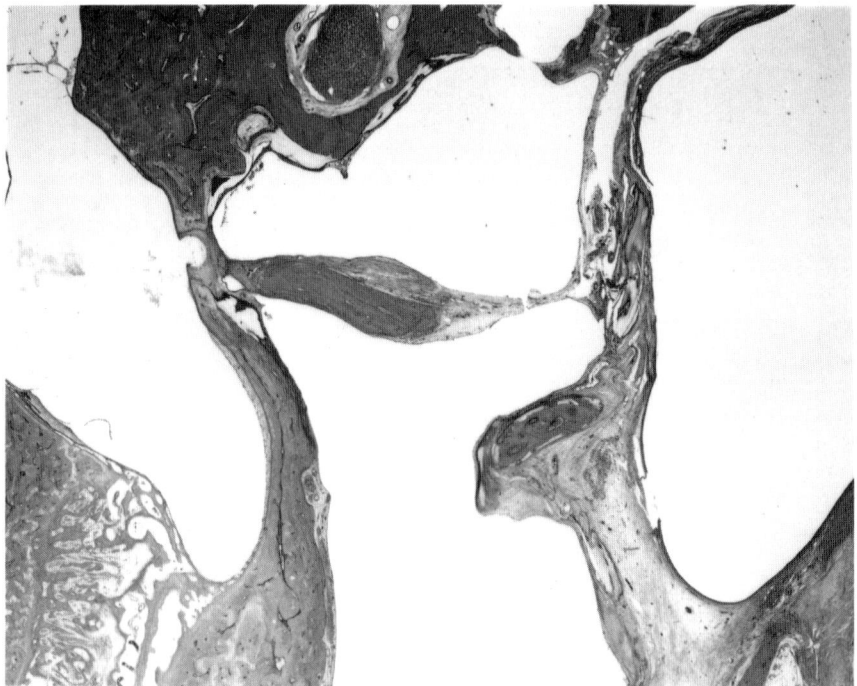

Figure 8.12. Fibrous thickening on the posterior surface of the graft will be seen later to be continuous with the stapedius tendon.

Prefabricated Allograft Ossiculoplasty 63

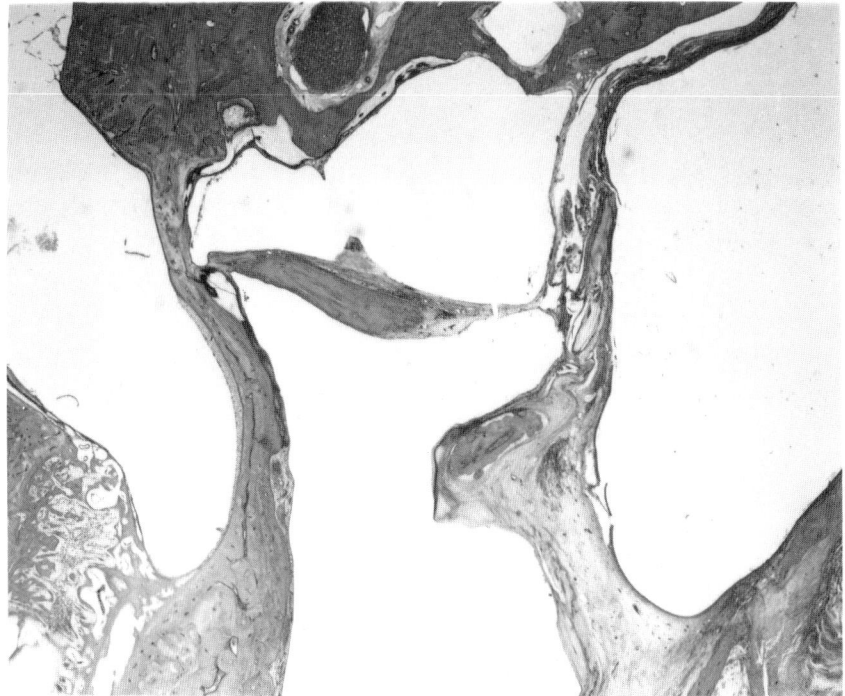

Figure 8.13. The stapedius tendon is seen now attached to the graft.

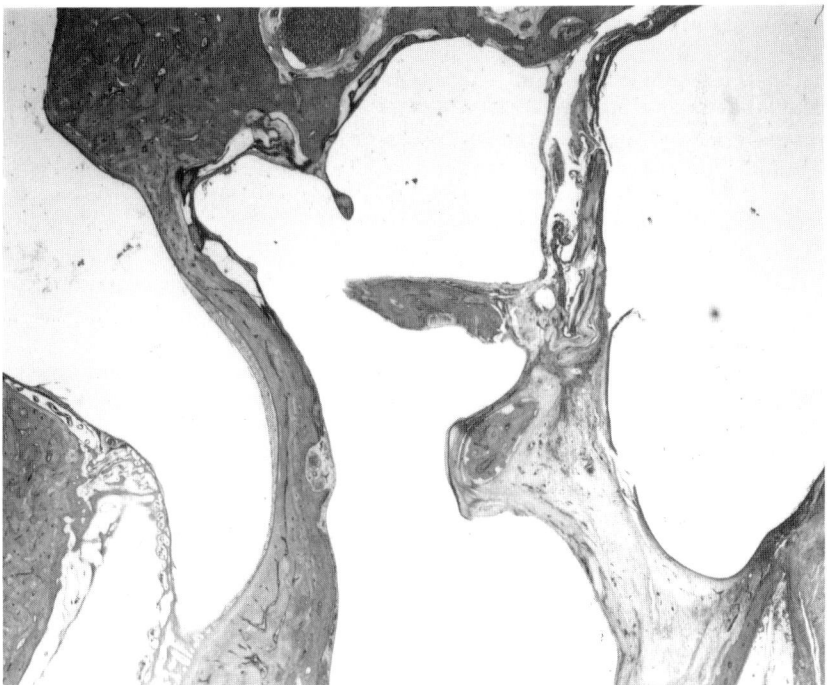

Figure 8.14. The tendon is near the posterior wall and this cut of the graft is also seen attached to the tympanic membrane by fibrous tissue.

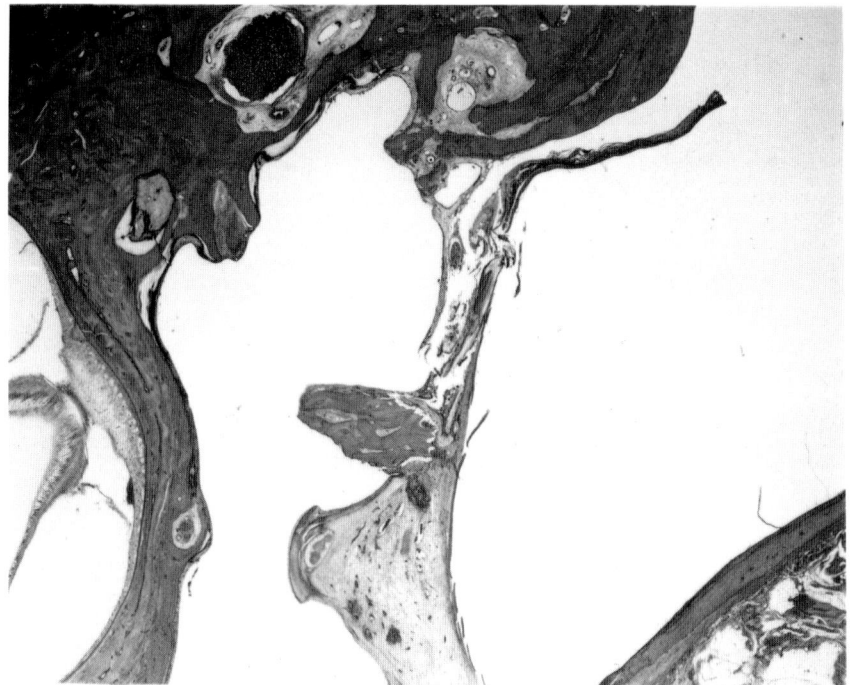

Figure 8.15. The bone allograft is seen embedded in the substance of the tympanic membrane as it has been serially followed across the middle ear. The tympanic membrane is considerably thickened by fibrous tissue and by a tympanosclerotic plaque on its middle ear surface.

lated directly to a malleal trough (1). The long range viability of these allografts is excellent.

Kerr (2) has pointed out that transplanted ossicles in animals show rapid replacement by new bone, a process called "creeping substitution." The amount of new bone laid down in humans is variable. It is possible that the allograft will be replaced by the patient's own tissue.

Very few of our patients have required revision surgery. Nevertheless, we cannot be sure how long these unextruded allografts will continue to survive and how long these nonvital bones will remain structurally adequate to serve as acoustic "conductors" (3–6).

Similar questions must be raised regarding other columellar substitutes used from tympanic membrane to stapes or oval window. Kerr (7) reported studies on 16 proplast and 52 plastipore prostheses removed at revision surgery. The very number of such prostheses requiring removal is striking. Multinucleated foreign body giant cells were found in both types of prostheses. Fibrous tissue invasion was found to be more consistent and widespread in proplast prostheses. Although no macroscopic disintegration was reported in any of these removed prostheses, Kerr asks the question, "Is it wise to continue to use prostheses where there is such marked evidence of foreign body giant cell reaction and where there is the suggestion of breakdown of the prosthesis?"

This study of a single ossiculoplastic case is of interest from the point of view of the extruded piece of allograft columella as well as in the histological status of the excellently functioning remaining intratympanic columellar allograft.

There is need for more histological studies on surgically removed or postmortem

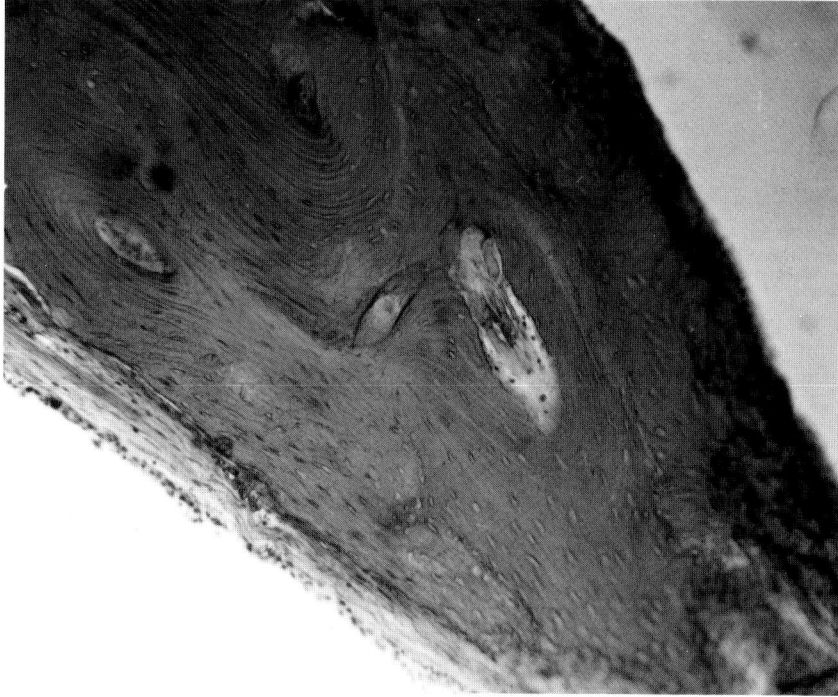

Figure 8.16. High power view. The bone allograft is almost completely acellular, except near the surface, in some regions, where small numbers of lacunae contain cells. The vascular channels within the bone, however, contain cells and these areas are continuous with cellular, fibrous tissue on the graft surface.

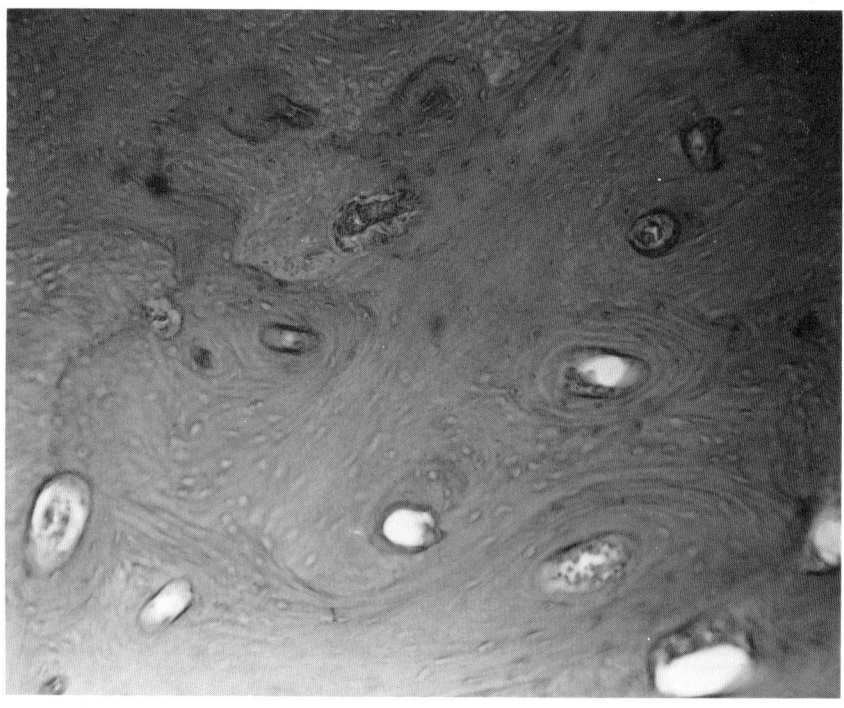

Figure 8.17. This is a normal incus section from a 78-year-old individual for comparison. One sees mostly empty lacunae, save for occasional perivascular regions where bone cells are present.

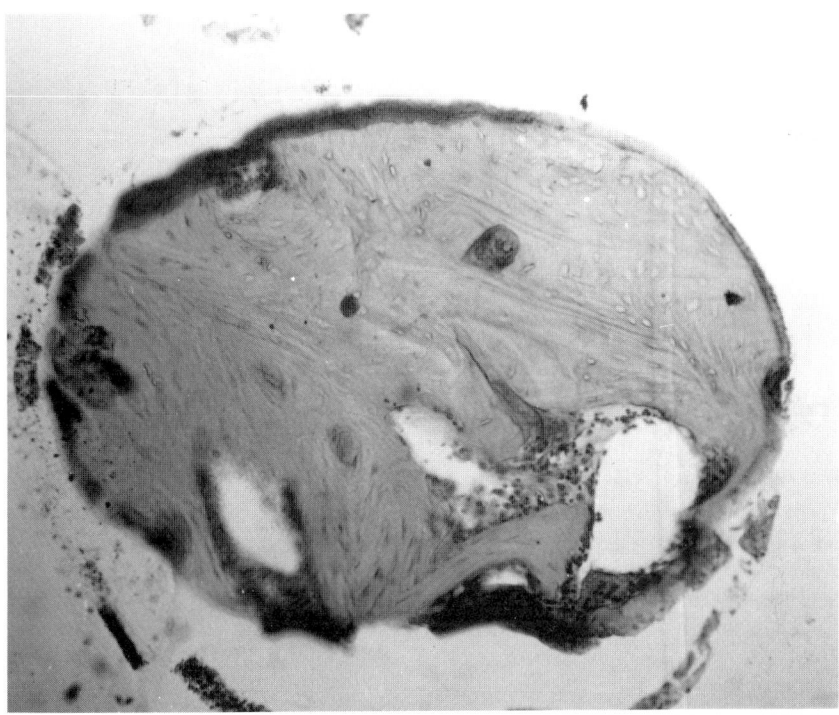

Figure 8.18. Postoperative exteriorized fragment of bone allograft is completely nonviable. No bone cells are evident. Small amounts of cellular fibrous tissue extend into the graft near the surface.

allograft and other ossicular substitutes. The long-range fate of all ossicular substitutes still remains an unknown.

References

1. Goodhill, V., Westerbergh, A.-M., and Davis, C. Prefabricated homografts in ossiculoplasty. *Trans Am Acad Ophthal Otolaryngol* 78: ORL 411-422, 1974.
2. Kerr, A.G. Homografts in middle ear. Letter to Editor. *J Roy Soc Med* 73: 610, 1980.
3. Smith, M.S.W., and Downey, D. Otologic Homograft indications, techniques and anatomic and functional results. *Trans Am Acad Ophthal Otolaryngol* 80: ORL 47-52, 1975.
4. Naujoks, J. Hornung, S., and Eitschberger, E. Eine klinische Studie uber allogenetische Ossikelimplantationen. *Laryngol Rhinol Otol* 57: 114-119, 1978.
5. Savary, P. La banque d'oreilles—difficultes et resultats. *J Otolaryng* 9: 177-183, 1980.
6. Ironside, W.M.S. Homograft ossicular reconstruction. *J Laryng Otol* 93: 1055-1061, 1979.
7. Kerr, A.G. Proplast and plastipore. *Clin Otolaryng* 6: 187-191, 1981.

CHAPTER 9

Tympanoplasty: Postoperative Retraction Pockets and Residual Cholesteatoma

James L. Sheehy, M.D.

You can avoid most problems in the management of chronic otitis media by not operating on ears without cholesteatoma and by performing a classical radical mastoidectomy (i.e., without functional reconstruction) on ears with cholesteatoma. But few would agree with this philosophy.

If you have the dual objectives of elimination of disease *and* functional reconstruction, you are faced with a dilemma, regardless of how you manage the mastoid when mastoidectomy is indicted. The more persistent you are in obtaining a good functional result, the more problems you may have. The problems are residual cholesteatoma and postoperative retraction pockets which may develop into cholesteatoma.

DEFINITIONS

Residual cholesteatoma is squamous epithelium not removed from the tubotympanic cleft at the time of cholesteatoma surgery (1). The surgeon may have left the cholesteatoma inadvertently or on purpose. We believe residual disease is an inherent problem in tympanoplasty for cholesteatoma, at least in the mesotympanum, regardless of the technique used in management of the mastoid (2).

Postoperative tympanic membrane retraction pockets, in contrast, need little in the way of definition. Although most commonly associated with cases of cholesteatoma managed by the intact canal wall (ICW) technique (in which it is properly called a recurrent cholesteatoma), they may occur following any reconstructive procedure on a patient with chronic otitis media.

There are three causes for postoperative retraction pockets (1): adhesions between the tympanic membrane and structures medial to it, Eustachian tube dysfunction, or atrophy of the reconstructed tympanic membrane followed by atelectasis. Postoperative retraction pockets are preventable (2).

SURGICAL PHILOSOPHY

A key factor in the interpretation and understanding of the incidence of postoperative retraction pockets and of residual cholesteatoma is an understanding of the surgeon's philosophy. Does he perform a tympanoplasty (functional reconstruction) on 90% or more of his cases, regardless of the extent of the mucous membrane disease or cholesteatoma? Or does he decide that a classical radical mastoidectomy is the procedure of choice in the most badly diseased ears? If he does perform tympanoplasty in cases with badly diseased middle ears, does he stage the operation in an attempt to obtain an air-containing mucosal-lined middle ear space? Or does he merely hope for the best with one operation?

The surgeon who performs a classical radical mastoidectomy (i.e., without functional reconstruction) on those cases with a destroyed middle ear will have effectively eliminated these cases from consideration of tympanoplasty results. He should have satisfactory functional results in many of the remaining (simpler) cases and should not be plagued by a high incidence of postoperative retraction pockets or of residual cholesteatoma.

The surgeon who does perform a tympanoplasty on the majority of his cases with a destroyed middle ear, but does not stage the operation to obtain an air-containing mucosal-lined middle ear space, may blame his functional failures and postoperative retraction pockets on a Eustachian tube problem. Palva, who apparently does not stage the operation, indicated in Tel-Aviv (3) that over one-third of his tympanoplasty cases had a nonfunctioning Eustachian tube postoperatively, compared with a 4% incidence in our experience (2).

The surgeon who performs tympanoplasty on almost all of his cholesteatoma cases, using the ICW technique, and who does not stage the operation, frequently will have a high incidence of recurrent cholesteatoma (postoperative retraction pockets) due to the formation of fibrous adhesions. He will have a low incidence of residual disease because it is not identified, at least early. This was true in our experience prior to 1967 (1) when we encountered recurrent cholesteatoma in over 20% of our cases and identified residual cholesteatoma in less than 10%. Now, with staged operations, the percentages are reversed: less than 5% recurrent cholesteatoma and over 20% with residual cholesteatoma in the middle ear (2).

OUR PHILOSOPHY

My philosophy, and the philosophy of my associates at the Otologic Medical Group, in the management of chronic ear disease is to obtain as safe an ear as possible, a dry ear, a hearing ear, and an ear that will require as little care as possible over the years. Management may or may not involve surgery.

Ears without cholesteatoma that are dry 99% of the time do not require surgery and the patient should be so informed. The safest thing for the patient to do is not to have surgry. If there is a hearing problem, a hearing aid is a very satisfactory solution.

If the patient wishes to have surgery or there is otorrhea or cholesteatoma, then the problem starts. Our objective is to obtain an ear free of disease with as good a functional result as possible, without needlessly creating an open mastoid cavity and the problems which may be involved with this cavity.

Accomplishing those objectives in the case of a dry central perforation with normal mucous membrane usually presents no difficulty, regardless of the ossicular chain problem involved. When there is considerable mucous membrane disease, or cholesteatoma, or both, accomplishing the dual objectives of a disease-free ear and a good functional result frequently requires a two-stage procedure. Residual cholesteatoma may be encountered, and one must take the necessary precautions to prevent postoperative retraction pockets, with recurrent cholesteatoma.

POSTOPERATIVE RETRACTION POCKETS

A retraction pocket into the middle ear (and epitympanum and mastoid) may develop in any patient, even those who have not had surgery. Is not that the way that cholesteatoma develops at times? The dynamics involved are similar in all cases. Because the major concern with postoperative retraction pockets is in cases in which an ICW procedure has been performed (regardless of whether there was cholesteatoma at the primary surgery), I will limit my further comments to postoperative retraction pockets in the ICW procedure: recurrent cholesteatoma (2). These comments involve development, avoidance, prevention, and treatment of postoperative retraction pockets.

Development

Four factors may be involved with the development of recurrent cholesteatoma: 1) an intact bony canal wall; 2) defects in the bone; 3) adhesions between the reconstructed tympanic membrane and the medial wall of the middle ear (and epitympanum and facial recess); 4) and Eustachian tube dysfunction. One may avoid the problem, prevent the problem, or treat it once it has developed.

Avoidance

The simplest way to avoid recurrent cholesteatoma is by not performing a tympanoplasty at all; limit cholesteatoma surgery to a classical radical mastoidectomy. One may minimize the complication in tympanoplasty by totally exteriorizing all mastoid cavities: do not perform an ICW procedure. Should tympanic membrane retraction occur, it will be limited to the middle ear and probably be attributed to malfunction of the Eustachian tube.

Those who prefer the ICW procedure in cholesteatoma surgery have learned that it may be wise to take the canal wall down in certain instances to prevent reoccurrence of cholesteatoma: 1) there is a long-standing serous otitis media in the other ear (in an adult); 2) the disease has caused a large defect in the canal wall; or 3) at the time of surgery it becomes apparent that it will be impossible to obtain an air-containing mucosal-lined middle ear space (rare).

Prevention

Those who use the ICW procedure to avoid an open mastoid cavity have learned that prevention is the key to success and that to prevent this complication one must do three things (4): 1) stage the operation in badly diseased ears; 2) repair defects in the canal wall; and 3) recognize Eustachian tube problems and ventilate the middle ear.

Staging the operation. Staging the operation is the key to success in the functional reconstruction in many cases of chronic otitis media (5). We do this to obtain a well-healed middle ear, an air-containing mucosal-lined middle ear space. Although staging may be indicated in only 10% of tympanoplasties without mastoidectomy, it is frequently indicated in badly diseased ears, with or without cholesteatoma.

Staging is indicated to prevent recurrent cholesteatoma which may develop as a result of a retraction pocket from fibrous adhesions between the reconstructed tympanic membrane and the middle ear, epitympanum, and facial recess. Staging, and the proper use of thick plastic, can avoid these adhesions.

Repair of canal wall defects. Even with proper staging, a retraction pocket can develop if a defect in the bone (usually the scutum) is not repaired at the second stage (4). We usually repair defects with cartilage and use cartilage routinely under the posterior superior part of the tympanic membrane in ossicular chain reconstruction with TORPs and PORPs.

Ventilation of the middle ear. Recurrent cholesteatoma can develop from a retraction pocket arising as a result of Eustachian tube dysfunction. Long-term transtympanic ventilation has been necessary in 4% of our ICW cases in the past (2).

Use of cartilage. We began using TORPs and PORPs routinely in functional reconstruction of the sound-pressure-transfer mechanism, always with a large piece of cartilage between the platform of the prosthesis and the tympanic membrane, in 1976 (6). Since then, it has become apparent that we, by so doing, were taking one more precaution to avoid postoperative retraction. The cartilage effectively blocks the area where these pockets usually occur.

Treatment

We recently reviewed 307 revision operations in 272 ICW cases (7). The majority were planned second-stage procedures within 2 years of the primary surgery. Thirty-eight, originally operated over a 20-year period, had recurrent cholesteatoma. Ten of the 38 were managed by a canal wall-down technique (Table 9.1).

The decision in such cases is based on two factors: 1) extent of canal wall destruction and 2) Eustachian tube function. If there is considerable canal wall destruction, we will create a cavity, and often obliterate with a Palva flap and bone paté

Table 9.1
Final Operative Procedure in 272 Patients whose Initial Operation was an ICW Procedure

Final Procedures	All Cases	Residual Found	Recurrent Present
Cavity created	13 (5%)	3 (4%)	10 (26%)
Canal wall reconstructed	5 (2%)	1 case	4 (10%)

(8). If the canal wall destruction is minimal, and Eustachian tube function seems adequate, reconstruction of the canal wall should be successful, with little risk of redevelopment of the retraction pocket.

If, on the other hand, there is a persistent Eustachian tube problem, regardless of the fact that there may be little canal wall destruction, we will take down the canal wall to prevent reoccurrence of the retraction pocket should the Eustachian tube dysfunction persist.

RESIDUAL CHOLESTEATOMA

We believe that residual cholesteatoma is unavoidable if one vigorously pursues a good functional result in all of his cholesteatoma surgery. Residual cholesteatoma was detected in 21% of 272 ears in a recent review (7).

Planned Revision

Residual cholesteatoma was suspected in one-half of the ears undergoing a planned first revision, but found in only 25%. Residual disease was more common in patients under age 16.

In those 153 cases in which the mastoid, epitympanum, and middle ear were re-explored at the time of the planned second stage, residual disease, suspected in two-thirds, was found in only one-third. Residua were more commonly found in the middle ear than in either the epitympanum or mastoid. A mastoid residuum was found in 10% and was the only location in two cases (Table 9.2).

The overall incidence of residual disease and the incidence by location was lower than we had previously reported (5). This is the result of having staged (re-explored) a higher percentage of primary cases, the majority of which did not have residual disease.

Unplanned Revisions

Two of the 28 ears in which both the middle ear and mastoid were re-explored at an unplanned revision had residual cholesteatoma. In neither case did this involve the mastoid.

CONCLUDING REMARKS

The incidence of postoperative problems in tympanoplasty surgery relates directly to the philosophy of the surgeon in selection both of patients and of operative procedures. The more vigorously one pursues a good functional result in all cases, the more problems he may encounter. These problems are postoperative retraction pockets (recurrent cholesteatoma) and residual cholesteatoma.

Postoperative retraction pockets are preventable in most cases. But this requires a two-stage procedure in badly diseased ears.

Residual cholesteatoma is unavoidable in badly diseased ears if one attempts to obtain an air-containing mucosal-lined middle ear space, for later functional reconstruction, in all cases.

The dual objectives in tympanoplasty

Table 9.2
Residual Disease in Planned and Unplanned First Revisions of ICW Cases in which Choleseteatoma was Present at the Initial Surgery and the Mastoid and Middle Ear were Re-Explored

Revisions	Residual Suspected	Residual Found	Location of Residua		
			Middle Ear	Epitympanum	Mastoid
Planned (125)	63%	33%	23%	18%	10%
Unplanned (28)		2 cases	1 case	1 case	
All cases	52%	28%	20%	15%	8%

surgery are to obtain an ear permanently free of disease and an ear with a good functional result. A planned two-stage procedure frequently will be required to accomplish these objectives.

References

1. Sheehy, J.L., and Patterson, M.E. Intact canal wall tympanoplasty with mastoidectomy: A review of 8 years experience. *Laryngoscope* 77: 1502–1542, 1967.
2. Sheehy, J.L., Brackmann, D.E., and Graham, M.D. Cholesteatoma surgery: Residual and recurrent disease: A review of 1024 cases. *Ann Otol Rhinol Laryngol* 86: 451–462, 1977.
3. Presentation of International Cholesteatoma Conference, Tel-Aviv, March, 1981.
4. Sheehy, J.L. Intact canal wall tympanoplasty with mastoidectomy. In *Controversy in Otolaryngology*, Snow, J.L. (Ed)., W.B. Saunders, Philadelphia, 1980, pp. 213–222.
5. Sheehy, J.L., and Crabtree, J.A. Tympanoplasty: staging the operation. *Laryngoscope* 83: 1594–1621, 1973.
6. Brackmann, D.E., and Sheehy, J.L. Tympanoplasty: TORPs and PORPs. *Laryngoscope* 89: 108–114, 1979.
7. Sheehy, J.L., and Robinson, J.V. Cholesteatoma surgery at the Otologic Medical Group, residual and recurrent disease. A report of 307 revision operations. *Am J Otol* (in publication).
8. Sheehy, J.L. Bone paté collecting device. *Otolaryngol Head Neck Surg* 88: 472, 1980.

CHAPTER 10

Management of Open, Diseased Mastoid Cavity

Tauno Palva, M.D.

INTRODUCTION

During the first part of the 20th century, surgery of a chronic middle ear disease consisted of two main operations. The modified radical mastoidectomy was employed for less infected cases with moderate tissue damage, while radical mastoidectomy was used in ears with severe middle ear cleft infection combined with extensive tissue alterations. It is quite understandable that our predecessors developed these open cavity operations because without antibiotics, all present day reconstructive tympanoplasties in these ears would have been doomed to failure. The disease was present in the form of active osteomyelitis, or cholesteatoma, or both, and leaving traces of either one in a closed middle ear or attic would have led to complications, often intracranial, in many of the ears.

However, there were some surgeons who foresaw that even without antibiotics, the operative procedure could be somewhat improved for the mastoid part of the operation. First of these is Mosher (1) who, in 1911, designed a superiorly based soft tissue flap from the postauricular area with a purpose for partial cavity obliteration. In 1935, Popper (2) utilized a meatally based thin periosteum flap to cover the raw bone surfaces in the cavity to aid in its epithelialization. Meurman and Ojala (3) tried to partially obliterate the cavity by utilizing an inferiorly based sternomastoid flap, swung to the lower part of the cavity. None of these operations became popular and until 1955, the open cavity method was used globally.

The technique my generation used in the post-Second World War period was an endaural approach in which the posterior meatal skin sleeve was at the end turned down to the cavity and fixed with catgut postauricularly. This served two purposes, by directing the skin flap to grow directly towards the cavity, and by enlarging the meatus considerably by turning posteriorly the endaural incision margins. I also covered the remaining raw bone surfaces with split-thickness skin grafts, as was the custom in many clinics, but suspected that epithelialization really occurred from the in-turned meatal skin.

RISING CRITICISM TOWARDS OPEN CAVITY SURGERY

During the 1950's, there were a few studies on the results of chronic ear surgery with the open cavity and some criticism arose against the method. In our own series (4, 5), the analyses showed that about 10% of the ears discharged continuously and in about 20%, there was intermittent moisture and the ears needed treatment three to four times annually. These figures were not at all bad as compared with several other series from the same period (6). Simson Hall's article from 1957 may be cited as one example of the troubles with open cavities, the finding being that 11% of the fenestration cavities for otosclerosis were wet or discharging.

I remember well sharing with the patient the dissatisfaction for ear surgery that had been made at the Department if the ear discharged continuously after surgery. This was particularly distressing if preoperatively the discharge had been scanty and not troublesome. The patient was told that it was better to have the pus coming out than to have it making its way in but

I had a nagging feeling that this was not really true and that something was at fault with the surgical method.

What was it then that went wrong in 10% of the cases definitely and in the 20% at least partially? Thinking about it now in retrospect, after more than 30 years experience in chronic ear surgery, several causes can be pointed out. One thing was the lack of a drill with different burr sizes to enable eradication of inflammatory changes in the perilabyrinthine bone and another, a much greater lack was that of magnification especially for the attic and middle ear cleft areas. One simply could not do present day thorough surgery in all cases, and the lack of antibiotics against pseudomonas and proteus infection added to these technical shortcomings. However, I think that these causes applied only to a limited number of these discharging ears. The main reason probably was that surgery was not thorough enough but tissue that could have been removed even with chisels and unaided eye was left behind and infection continued producing granulating sick cavities. The sigmoid and dural lamina were not always chiselled down to healthy thin bone, and granulating air cells were sometimes left in the Trautmann's triangle and to the epitympanum. There was no systematic teaching in ear surgery at that time and many surgeons did this work with minimal anatomic knowledge.

With this background, the more ambitious among the specialty drew their conclusions in the latter part of 1950's and, provided with burrs, microscopes, and antibiotics, thought that it was time to eradicate the disease totally and try to reconstruct the tympanic cavity and the posterior ear canal and, thus, to get rid of the cavity altogether. My own basic line has been canal wall down with eradication of disease, canal wall reconstruction, and mastoid obliteration, even if I have given a passing try to some other methods like the canal up procedure running high with the tide. The method developed suits exceptionally well the management of open diseased mastoid cavities.

However, before I start discussing the surgical treatment, I wish to point out that the open cavity method is, in less experienced hands, certainly much safer than the canal wall up procedure. In Helsinki clinic before my time, from 1974, ear surgery was not the main interest area and the ability and knowledge in this field can be said to have been at the average level for otolaryngologists. My associate, Palmgren, studied 183 cases operated during the years 1964-1968 by the open method without reconstruction, cholesteatoma being present in 143 (78%). The average observation time was 10 years, the maximum 42 and minimum 6 years. There was discharge from the cavities in 22% while in 10%, the cavity was subjectively dry but there was moisture under the crust removed once or twice yearly. Thus, 68% of the cavities were troublefree. The figure for recurrent cholesteatoma was as low as 6.3% which is quite superior to the figures reported by most experienced ear surgeons using the canal wall up procedure.

MANAGEMENT OF DISEASED OPEN CAVITIES

When the patient presents in the office with a discharging open radical cavity, the surgeon should ask himself: can this ear be brought to a dry state with conservative means alone or is a reconstructive procedure with obliteration necessary? This can be answered generally during the first visit: if there are granulations all over the cavity, the indication for revision surgery is obvious. Histologically, behind this granulation tissue, there will always be areas with infected bone that has to be drilled off before a dry state can be hoped for. However, in some cases, there are only one or two small granulating areas, while the cavity skin in other areas is healthy. These ears can be treated conservatively in the office: local anesthesia is provided with Bonain solution in a cottonoid and the granulation tissue with the adjoining granulating air cells is scraped clean with a sharp curette under microscopic control. Painting the surfaces with 0.5% gentianviolett cures, the infection and skin from the surroundings rapidly grows in to cover the raw surfaces. A new operation should be offered to those patients only if there is evidence of a satisfactory Eustachian tube function to guarantee a successful tympanoplasty.

Once the decision to reoperate the more extensively diseased cases has been made, bacterial culture is made for identification and sensitivity testing. This should never be omitted because it is essential to know which antibiotic should be used in connection with surgery. There are three bacterial strains that make up 95% of cavity bacteria, viz. pseudomonas, proteus strains, and staphylococci. For pseudomonas, there was a time when gentamycin and colimycin were the only effective antibiotics but recently, we have found several cases resistant to gentamycin but sensitive to trimetoprim-sulfa combination or to chloramphenicol. The effective drug used in the treatment should be known in advance as well as its cost to the patient.

I have found the application of gentian violet into the cavity and middle ear to be the most effective presurgical means in diminishing or even temporarily abating the infection. In addition, the cavity part is filled with gentamycin-vaselin, injected in place with a 2-ml syringe through a curved, large-bore suction tip. If a decision to use ototoxic drops is made, the patient should be observed once weekly and the drops discontinued as soon as the discharge starts to clearly abate. I have seen several ears in which continued use of ototoxic drops in a dry ear has led to permanent deafness.

SURGICAL PROCEDURE

The ears are always operated by using the postauricular approach, an incision being made 2-3 cm posterior to the postauricular fold. Skin is undermined posteriorly and a large musculoperiosteal flap is created, its size being estimated by the size of the open mastoid cavity. The flap is dissected towards the auricle, care being taken not to open the cavity at this stage. Opening would endanger the collection of sterile bone patè.

Using the largest possible cutting burr, continuous irrigation and low power suction, cortical bone is drilled on top of the sigmoid sinus, on the bone lateral to the middle fossa, on the zygomatic region, and collected.

The development of the musculoperiosteal flap is completed anteriorly and the cavity, containing a gentianviolet-soaked tamponade from previous evening, is opened.

It is quite seldom that the mastoid tip is found to have been removed during primary surgery, Periosteum covered bone chips, therefore can be chiselled off from it, the removed pieces being kept in an ampicillin solution until used, similar to bone patè.

The soft tissue lining of the cavity is next dissected with ear canal elevator and excised saving only enough skin inferiorly, superiorly, and laterally to provide a skin lining for the medial part of the ear canal. All skin and granulating tissue in the medial part of the cavity is removed up to the level of facial nerve canal.

In infected cavities, one generally finds a large overhang of the temporal dural lamina and sometimes even in the sigmoid sinus area. The lamina are exposed and followed down to the medial part of the cavity, initially posteriorly, along the sinodural angle. Here one nearly always finds granulating air cells, often extending deep into Trautmann's triangle. Drilling is done to the white, glistening lamellar bone. The superior semicircular canal is then identified and cell tracks on either side of it are drilled away with a diamond burr. On the superior side, one sometimes must remove the dural lamina also as the diseased bone does not allow leaving even a thin lamina. On the inferior side, in the Trautmann's triangle, drilling is continued until the air cells are removed and the blood vessels in the bone are encountered between the superior and posterior canals.

In some revision surgery ears, problems may arise because the cavity skin may be directly united with sigmoid sinus wall or temporal dura in those ears when the laminar bony wall has been removed. Excision of cavity skin in these areas should be done under microscopic control, using either a sharp ear canal elevator or a knife to cleanly separate the two tissues. I have not had any difficulty with the sinus wall and a small tear can always be easily repaired with cottonoid and fascia. In temporal dura areas, separation of skin from dura has necessitated, in several cases, dissection of part of the dural surface into the skin specimen in order to be sure of total removal of squamous epithelium. These weaker areas are subsequently covered by lyophilized dura and finally, obliteration removes all possibilities of a later herniation. If there is already herniation into the cavity, resection of the herniated area must be made using a middle fossa additional approach. Here again obliteration removes the difficulties with possible postoperative CSF leaks. However, this procedure should not be attempted by inexperienced surgeons but the cases should be referred to surgeons used to these approaches.

Cleaning of the mastoid tip generally is one of the easier tasks and distinct marrow bone need not be removed. In some ears, there are granulating air cells in the area close to the facial nerve, and posteromedial to it, and one has to proceed, if need be, even down to the jugular bulb. Surgery in this part is very similar to endolymphatic sac surgery and presents no difficulty to a well-trained surgeon.

Before proceeding to the tympanic work proper, the posterior lower ear canal wall is drilled away level with the inferior part of the ear canal. This bone practically always contains granulating air cells which, for a less experienced surgeon, may simulate the facial nerve. One has to keep the nerve canal continuously in sight and remember that the nerve does not make any odd slopes but continues directly from the anterior margin of the horizontal semicircular canal. Only in very sclerotic mastoids, the nerve is more superficial than one might expect and has to be watched for more carefully. Exposure of the pyramidal process and the stapedial muscle marks well the anterior margin of the facial nerve. The burr size here must be kept sufficiently small initially so that when one focusses on the inferior margin of the bridge, the upper edge of the burr must not touch the stapes head. Some of the unexpected sensorineural losses have their origin from this accident, often not even noted by the surgeon.

Attention is next turned to the epitympanic space, one of the areas where incompetent surgery is most often made. Because the temporal dural lamina bends medially, both osteomyelitic bone, or squamous epithelium, may be left into the shadow of the laminar overhang. The surgeon must start from the lateral part of the dural lamina and continue drilling medially along the lamina. The microscope has to be shifted caudally in order to provide a good view to the inbending lamina. My rule is that the surgeon must see the entire dural lamina from its lateral part down to the area of the geniculate ganglion. This standard procedure guarantees that all squamous epithelium can be removed from the epitympanum. Drilling is continued, if needed, under direct vision up to the orifice of the Eustachian tube.

The tympanic part of the surgery does not differ from the steps employed during primary surgery in chronically discharging ears. In this patient material, one generally finds a large pars tensa defect, often combined with epidermization of the promontory. If there is good mucosa in the Eustachian tube orifice, with an air bubble seen during the nitrous oxide phase of the anesthesia, ossicular reconstruction from the stapes head or from the footplate may give excellent hearing results. If the Eustachian tube is blocked by fibrous tissue and the other ear is normal, I see no point in taking exaggerated pains to create an aerated tympanic cavity. In all cases, however, I will do the tympanic reconstruction, because this may affect favorably the phase shift between the oval and round windows and give reasonably good hearing even in adhesive middle ears. All squamous epithelium must be removed from the tympanic cleft and for me, this means removal of most of the inflamed mucosa. This is based on the tympanic biopsies that I routinely take from different areas; these have in 10–15% demonstrated squamous epithelium in areas that, in the operative notes, were judged nonsquamous.

All raw surfaces in the tympanic cleft should be covered before reconstruction. To this purpose, I have found the thin sheets of lyophilized dura best, dissected by the nurse during surgery. This tissue, when thin enough, conforms well to the noneven surfaces of the tympanic cavity, especially in the hypotympanum where diamond drill may have been used extensively to remove the disease from the pericochlear cells. In a few months time, this dura will be transformed into normal mucosa, growing from the Eustachian tube.

I have found that reconstruction from the footplate should be made with a homograft incus, the short process of which rests on the footplate, part of the body is trimmed, and the long process rests on a piece of lyophilized dura in the orifice of the Eustachian tube. This is covered first with a thin dura lying on the annular bone, with a hole cut into it on the highest part of the prosthesis. This aids the surgeon to see that the prosthesis has kept its proper place and effectively stabilizes it. Fascia is then used to cover the dura in a double-layer fashion and the meatal skin adjusted on top of the fascial margins.

Obliteration of the cavity is made in the routine fashion. Bone paté is pressed dry and cemented to the cavity, starting from Trautmann's triangle and filling most of the cavity. Anteriorly filling extends to the facial canal area where the paté is covered with bone chips and possibly with lyophilized dura. The tympanic membrane level is supported with small gauze strips while the meatus is filled with gentamycin, vaselin impregnated gauze. The inferior, superior, and lateral cavity skin remnants are turned posterior to the gauze, and the remaining part of the fascia lifted up to cover them from the posterior side. The epitympanic space is filled with pieces of lyophilized dura, bone paté, and bone chips and the musculoperiosteal flap is turned down to obliterate the cavity. If part of an initially large cavity still needs filling, the remaining bone paté and bone chips are employed to fill the empty spaces. This is followed by inserting the drain and suturing the wound.

The results of this surgery are very gratifying. In a series of 80 cases with continuous discharge in all before surgery, all except one are dry and this one patient needs treatment two to three times a year. I have suggested revision surgery for her because she initially had a very large cavity and I did not fill it sufficiently well. However, she considers the present status to be good and has declined further surgery. In another patient, heavily radiated because of uvular carcinoma, discharge persisted until the death, and he needed treatment every 2 months.

The average preoperative hearing for the three middle frequencies was 58.5 dB and as an average for 3 years postoperatively was 42 dB. There are several ears with hearing up to 20-dB level all of whom had Eustachian tube with normal mucosa; in 30 ears altogether the tympanic membrane was mobile postoperatively. The majority, 50 ears, showed adhesive changes and the hearing remained around 50-60 dB.

In summary, there is no better method for surgery of the open, diseased cavity than the obliteration method described (8, 9). It consistently produces dry ears and near-normal ear canals. The ossicular chain and tympanic membrane can be reconstructed according to the common principles and in cases with a functioning Eustachian tube, good hearing results can be expected.

References

1. Mosher, H.P. A method of filling the excavated mastoid with a flap from the back of the auricle. *Laryngoscope* 21: 1158-1163, 1911.
2. Popper, O. Periosteal flap grafts in mastoid operation. *S Afr Med J* 9: 77-78, 1935.
3. Meurman, Y., and Ojala, L. Primary reduction of large operation cavity in radical mastoidectomy with a muscle. *Acta Otolaryngol (Stockh)* 37: 245-252, 1949.
4. Palva, T., and Pulkkinen, K. Hearing after surgery in chronically discharging ears. I. *Acta Otolaryngol (Stockh)* 51: 123-134, 1960.
5. Palva, T., and Pulkkinen, K. Hearing after surgery in chronically discharging ears. II. *Acta Otolaryngol (Stockh)* 52: 175-185, 1960.
6. Beales, P.H. The problem of the mastoid segment after tympanoplasty. *J Laryngol Otol* 73: 527-531, 1959.
7. Hall, I.S. The mobilization operation in the treatment of otosclerosis. *J Laryngol Otol* 72: 93-100, 1958.
8. Palva, T. Operative technique in mastoid obliteration. *Acta Otolaryngol (Stockh)* 75: 289-290, 1973.
9. Palva, T., and Mäkinen, J. The meatally based musculoperiosteal flap in cavity obliteration. *Arch Otolaryngol* 105: 377-380, 1979.

CHAPTER 11
Stapedotomy versus Stapedectomy

Ugo P. Fisch, M.D.

The number of operations performed for the treatment of otosclerosis is declining throughout the world. Because of this, the experience accumulated by the individual otological surgeon with stapedectomy is also decreasing. Therefore, it is justified to pursue the development of an operative technique which will be simple and result in the lowest postoperative complication rate.

At present, otosclerosis is approached surgically in two divergent ways. Total or subtotal removal of the stapes footplate (stapedectomy) with tissue graft sealing of the oval window is still considered the best guarantee against postoperative fistula formation by many otologists. On the other hand, recent reports by Marquet et al. (1) and Smyth and Hassard (2) indicate that limited opening (0.3–0.7 mm) of the stapes footplate (stapedotomy) significantly reduces the risk of immediate and delayed inner ear deafness (Fig. 11.1).

From the theoretical point of view, stapedotomy offers several advantages over stapedectomy. A limited hole into the stapes footplate limits the possibility of a direct lesion of the cochlear duct, saccule, and utricle. In this regard, the investigation of 30 normal temporal bones of our histological collection revealed that the utricle is attached to the superior half of the footplate in two-thirds of the cases. This situation (Fig. 11.2) defies the most careful manipulations and may lead to inner ear damage following stapedectomy.

After stapedotomy, sudden movements of the long process of the incus have less effect on the inner ear or on the loop attachment of the prosthesis since they displace a much smaller volume of perilymph than after stapedectomy. Furthermore, stapedotomy prevents migration of the prosthesis induced by scarring in the oval window niche (3).

In order to find out whether the mentioned advantages of stapedotomy versus stapedectomy are real, the results obtained by the same surgeon with both techniques between 1970–1978 were analyzed.

RESULTS OF STAPEDOTOMY (0.6 MM WIRE TEFLON PISTON) VERSUS STAPEDECTOMY (WIRE CONNECTIVE TISSUE)

Of 340 consecutive primary operations performed between 1970–1978, 170 were total or partial stapedectomies and 170 stapedotomies. A self-manufactured wire connective tissue prosthesis was used in stapedectomy and a 0.6-mm wire teflon piston with venous blood sealing (3) for stapedotomy. Both groups of patients had

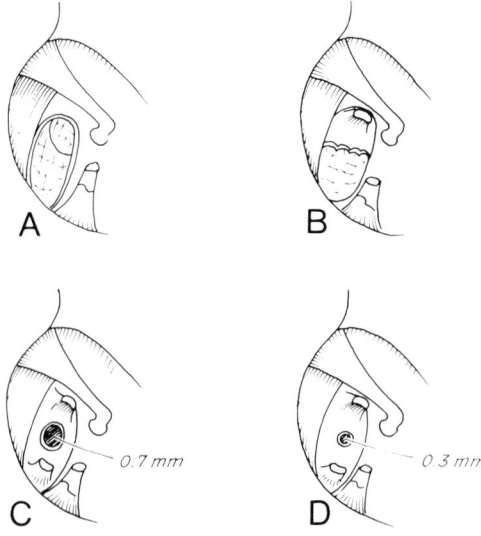

Figure 11.1. Total (*A*) or subtotal (*B*) stapedectomy versus stapedotomy (*C*, *D*).

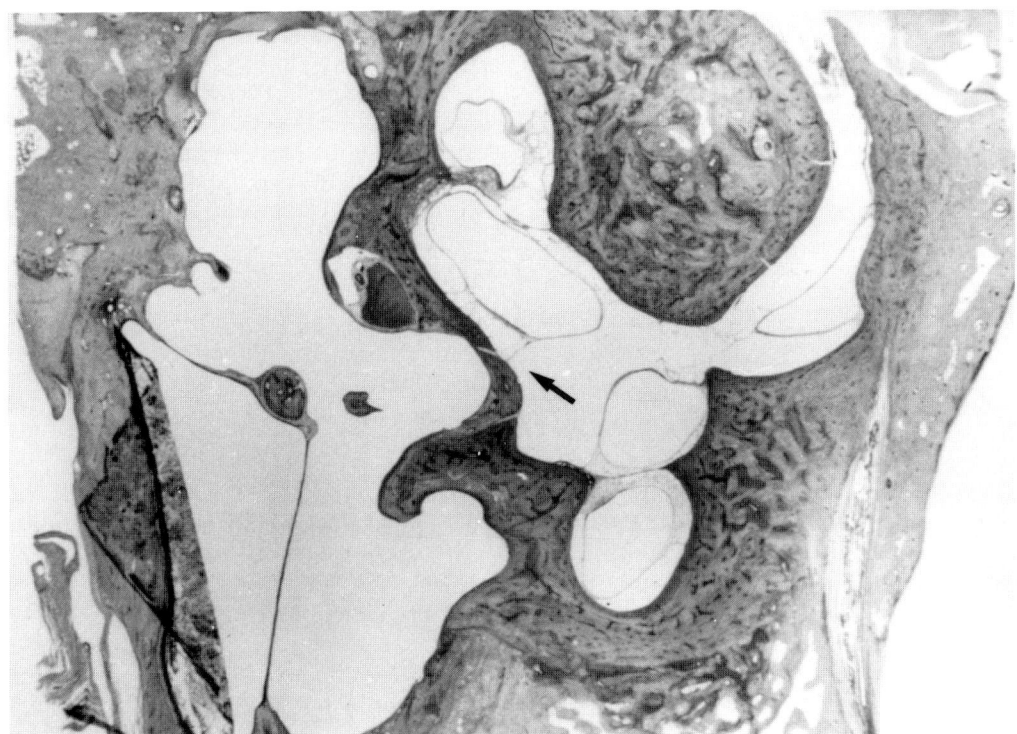

Figure 11.2. Fibrous attachment of the utricle to the upper half of the stapes. H.E., vertical cut through a normal temporal bone. U = utricle, S = saccule.

measurable hearing and were homogenous as far as age, sex and preoperative bone- and air-conduction levels were concerned. The follow-up study did not reveal any significant difference between the number of patients reaching the 0–5 dB or 0–10 dB airbone gap closure at 3 weeks, 3 months, 1 and 3 years after stapedectomy or stapedotomy (Tables 11.1 and 11.2). There was, however, a significant advantage in favor of stapedotomy (Table 11.3) when considering the gap between the preoperative bone conduction and postoperative air conduction at 4000 Hz 1 year postoperatively. The stapedotomy patients presented also with a higher bone conduction improvement and less impairement 3 years following surgery (Table 11.4). These findings confirm that stapedotomy is less traumatic to the inner ear than stapedectomy and are in agreement with those published by Smyth and Hassard (2). In contrast to the latter authors, we were unable to find any significant difference in the rate of immediate postoperative hearing losses occurring in both groups of patients (Table 11.5). The only dead ear observed in the presented 340 primary operations (0.3 %) occurred, however, after a plain stapedectomy.

In view of the better hearing resulting

Table 11.1
0–5 dB Postoperative Airborne Gap (0.5–2 kHz/3) for Stapedectomy (Connective Tissue Wire Prosthesis) and Stapedotomy (0.6-mm Wire Teflon Piston)

Follow-Up Time	Connective-Tissue Wire	Wire-Teflon Piston (0.6 mm)	P
3 weeks	23%	15%	NS
3 months	38%	28%	NS
1 year	31%	22%	<0.1
3 years	24%	33%	NS

Table 11.2
0–10 dB Postoperative Airborne Gap (0.5–2 kHz) for Stapedectomy (Connective Tissue Wire Prosthesis) and Stapedotomy (0.6 mm Wire Teflon Piston)

Follow-Up Time	Connective-Tissue Wire	Wire-Teflon Piston (0.6 mm)	P
3 weeks	44%	38%	NS
3 months	58%	51%	NS
1 year	54%	58%	NS
3 years	58%	52%	NS

Table 11.3
Airbone Gap at 4000 Hz (1 year postoperatively) for Stapedectomy (Connective Tissue Wire Prosthesis) and Stapedotomy (0.6-mm Wire Teflon Piston)

dB	Connective-Tissue Wire	Wire-Teflon Piston (0.6 mm)	P
Overclosure	12%	28%	<0.05
0–5	25%	49%	<0.05
0–10	44%	61%	<0.05

Table 11.4
Difference in Bone Conduction (3 years Postoperatively) between Stapedectomy (Connective Tissue Wire Prosthesis) and Stapedotomy (0.6-mm Wire Teflon Piston)

Type of Prosthesis	Improvement (10 dB or more)	Impairement (10 dB or more)
Connective-Tissue wire	0%	9%
Wire-Teflon piston	18%	0%
P	<0.05	<0.1

from stapedotomy in the higher frequency range and considering the fact that a limited fenestration with wire teflon piston proved as safe as the connective tissue graft sealing of the oval window, we decided to abandon total or subtotal stapedectomy in favor of stapedotomy. This decision was also influenced by the simplification resulting from the use of a prefabricated wire teflon piston instead of the self-made wire connective tissue prosthesis. The experience gained with stapedotomy made us aware that to create a small fenestra is not always as easy as advocated by its propagators particularly in presence of minimal otosclerotic anterior fixation. The cracks and fractures resulting from the conventional breaking off of the stapedial arch lead eventually to a subtotal stapedectomy preventing a limited footplate fenestration. Therefore, we came to the conclusion that consistent performance of stapedotomy is only possible if the conventional steps of stapes surgery are reversed and the desired opening into the footplate is performed *before* altering the integrity of the incudo-stapedial joint or of the stapes arch. Under these circumstances, the maximal diameter of limited footplate opening is of 0.5 mm. It was necessary therefore, to design a new 0.4 mm-wire teflon piston (Richards Manufacturing Co. Inc., Memphis, TN, USA) to accomodate into this opening.

Technique of Stapedotomy

The single steps of the 0.4-mm wire teflon piston stapedotomy technique are as follows (Fig. 11.3). The length of the prosthesis is first determined by measuring the distance between the stapes footplate and the lateral surface of the incus. To this latter measure, 0.25 mm is than added in order to account for the penetration into the vestibule (Fig. 11.3A). A three-edged manual trephine is then used to perform

Table 11.5
Immediate, Sensorineural Hearing Loss Following Stapedectomy (Connective Tissue Wire Prosthesis) and Stapedotomy (0.6-mm Wire Teflon Piston)

Type of Prosthesis	n	%
Connective-Tissue wire	1/170	0.6
Wire-Teflon piston (0.6 mm)	0/170	0*
All cases	1/340	0.3

* P = NS.

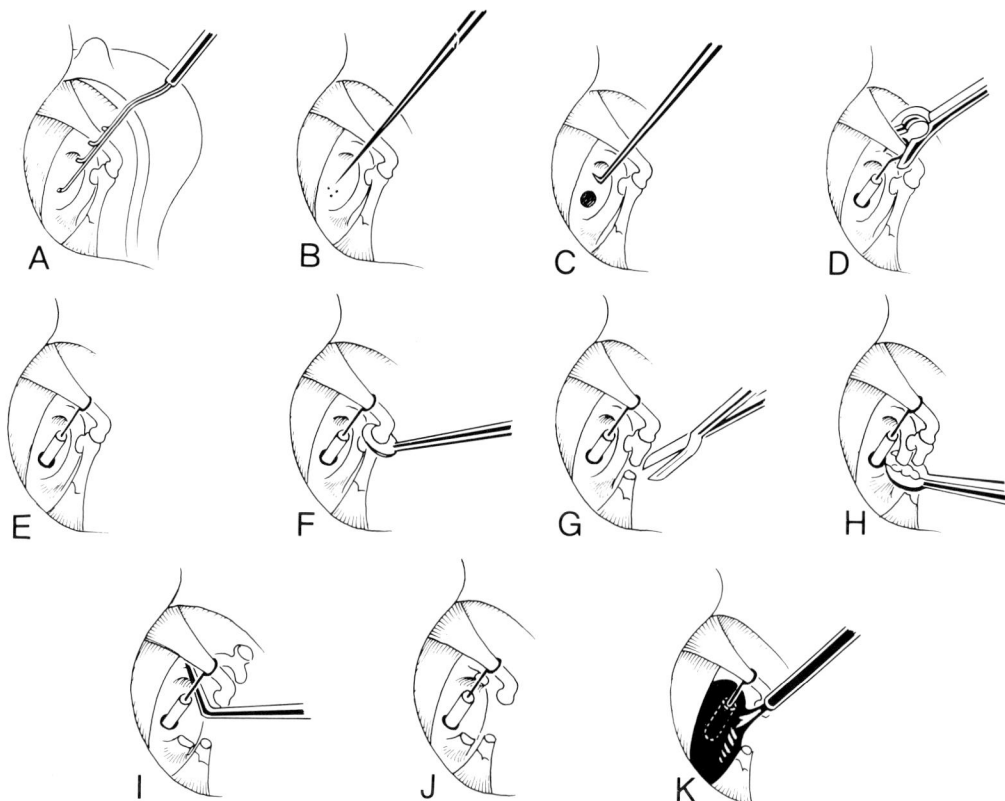

Figure 11.3. Technique of stapedotomy. A. determination of the length of the prosthesis. B. perforation of the visible, central portion of the footplate. C. creation of a 0.5-mm opening with the 0.2-mm right angle hook. D. the 0.4-mm wire piston is brought into position and articulated to the incus *before* violating the integrity of the incudo-stapedial joint and stapedial arch. Technique of stapedotomy. E. surgical site following placement of the 0.4-mm prosthesis. F. the incudo-stapedial joint is disrupted with a round knife. G. the stapedial tendon is cut with small tympanoplasty scissors. H. the stapes crura are severed with special crurotomy scissors. I. following section of the crura, the stapes arch is removed using a 1-mm 45° angle hook. J. surgical site following removal of the stapes arch. K. the stapedotomy opening is sealed with blood withdrawn from the cubital vein of the patient.

three small openings into the visible, central part of the footplate (Fig. 11.3B). The bone between the initial openings is removed with a 0.2-mm right angle hook. This instrument, that should be called shovel because of its broad tip, is also used to enlarge the fenestra to the desired diameter (Fig. 11.3C). A caliber rod assists in determining the definite size of the fenestra. At this moment the 0.4-mm wire teflon piston is brought into position and articulated to the incus with the help of a modified McGee crimper (Fig. 11.3D). The preservation of the integrity of the incudo-stapedial joint and stapedial arch permits to take advantage of the undisturbed natural fixation of the stapes, avoids hemorrhage and prevents undue movements of the incus when crimping the prosthesis on it. When the prosthesis is in place (Fig. 11.3E), the incudo-stapedial joint is disrupted with a round knife (Fig. 11.3F), the stapedial tendon is cut with small tympanoplasty scissors (Fig. 11.3G) and the stapes crura are severed with special crurotomy scissors (Fig. 11.3H). The separated stapes arch is removed with a 1-mm 45° angle hook (Fig. 11.3I). The use of crurotomy scissors avoids the uncontrolled trauma resulting from the conventional break-off of the stapes arch (Fig. 11.3J). Blood withdrawn from the cubital vein of the patient at the beginning of the operation is used to seal the stapedotomy opening at the end of the procedure (Fig. 11.3K). Only one size wire teflon piston is used. The 7-mm long prosthesis is trimmed to the desired length using a special cutting board (Richards Manufacturing Co. Inc., Memphis, TN, USA) (Fig. 11.4). The cutting board carries a 0.4-mm hole in which the prosthesis is stored until use. Storage of the prosthesis on the board helps to pick up the latter in the proper angle and simplifies therefore its placement.

Table 11.6
0–5 dB Postoperative Airbone Gap (0.5–2 kHz/3) after Stapedotomy with the 0.6-mm and 0.4-mm Wire Teflon Piston

Follow-Up Time	Wire-Teflon Piston 0.6 mm	Wire-Teflon Piston 0.4 mm	P
3 weeks	15%	0%	<0.05
3 months	28%	8%	<0.01
1 year	22%	9%	NS

Table 11.7
0–10 dB Postoperative Airbone Gap (0.5–2 kHz/3) after Stapedotomy with 0.6-mm and 0.4-mm Wire Teflon Piston

Follow-Up Time	Wire-Teflon Piston 0.6 mm	Wire-Teflon Piston 0.4 mm	P
3 weeks	38%	13%	<0.025
3 months	51%	36%	NS
1 year	58%	24%	<0.001

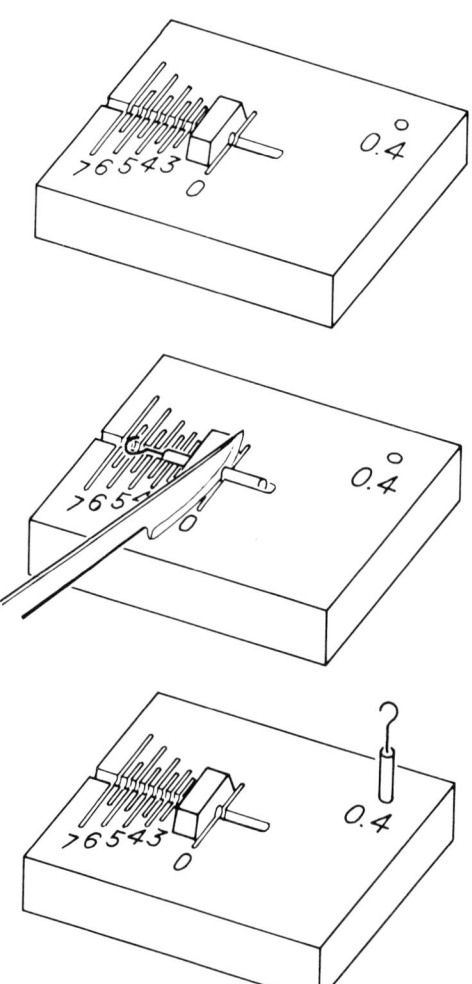

Figure 11.4. Cutting and storage board for the 0.4-mm wire teflon piston. Note that only one size wire teflon piston is used. The 7-mm long prosthesis is trimmed to the desired length.

RESULTS OF STAPEDOTOMY (0.4-MM VERSUS 0.6-MM WIRE TEFLON PISTON)

The first 52 patients operated according to the previously described technique between 1979 and 1980 having been followed for at least 1 year have been reviewed. Table 11.6 shows that there was no significant difference between the results of both prosthesis 1 year postoperatively although there were less patients with the 0.4-mm piston reaching a closure of the airbone gap of 5 dB or less 3 weeks and 3 months following surgery. This indicates that a smaller fenestra needs more time to reach a perfect success than a larger one. Considering the 0.10-dB airbone gap, the 0.4-mm piston yielded poorer results than the 0.6-mm piston at the 3 weeks' and 1 year's follow-up (Table 11.7). No statistical difference is found between the number of patients reaching the 0–10 dB airbone gap with the 0.6-mm wire teflon piston and those reaching the 0–15 dB gap with the 0.4-mm piston (Table 11.8). This means that for 0.5–2 kHz the results of the 0.4-mm piston are worse than those of the 0.6 mm piston but only for 5 dB. Smyth and Hassard (2) made a similar observation using the 0.3-mm all teflon piston. Marquet (3) has also demonstrated that stapedotomy results are not as good as those of stapedectomy in the lower frequencies.

This author, as well as Smyth and Hassard (2) advocate the use of small fenestras because of the better performance in the higher frequencies. This was also the case in our experience since, at 4000 Hz, equally good results were found 1 year postoperatively for both, the 0.4-mm and the 0.6-mm wire teflon piston (Table 11.9). The better hearing results in the higher frequencies and the smaller trauma to the inner ear are the factors that have prompted us to continue the experience with the 0.4-mm piston. A longer follow-up and a large number of cases are needed to decide whether the decreased hearing in the lower frequencies with the 0.4-mm piston is indeed permanent. Figure 11.5 shows that there is a tendency toward improvement in the low frequencies after 1 year. Smyth and Hassard (2) also have stated that the results of the 0.3-mm all teflon piston in the low frequency range improved to the level of those obtained with stapedectomy after 2–3 years.

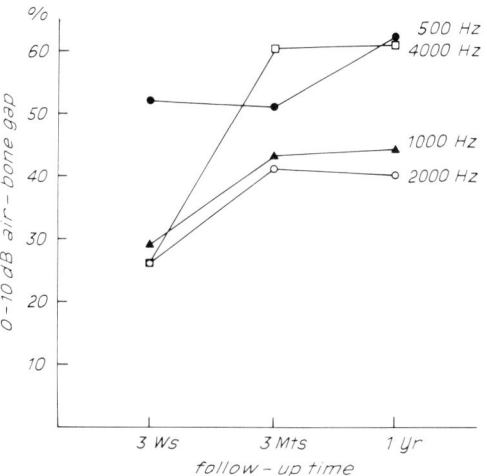

Figure 11.5. 0–10 dB airbone gap for the three response frequencies 3 weeks, 3 months, and 1 year following surgery. There is a tendency for improvement at the 1 year's follow-up. This is particularly true for the frequency of 500 Hz that is comparable with 4000 Hz 1 year postoperatively.

Table 11.8
Comparison between the 0–10 dB Airbone Gap for the 0.6-mm Wire Teflon Piston and the 0–15 dB Airbone Gap for the 0.4-mm Wire Teflon Piston (0.5–2 kHz/3)

Follow-Up Time	Wire-Teflon Piston 0.6 mm (0–10 dB)	Wire-Teflon Piston 0.4 mm (0–15 dB)	P
3 weeks	38%	32%	NS
3 months	51%	60%	NS
1 year	58%	56%	NS

Table 11.9
Airbone Gap at 4000 Hz (1 year postoperatively). Comparison of the Results of the 0.6-mm and 0.4-mm Wire Teflon Piston

dB	Wire-Teflon Piston 0.6 mm	Wire-Teflon Piston 0.4 mm	P
Overclosure*	28%	36%	NS
0–5	49%	45%	NS
0–10	61%	61%	NS

* Connective-tissue wire overclosure = 12%.

CONCLUSIONS

1. Stapedotomy with wire teflon piston does not increase the risk of postoperative fistula formation in comparison to stapedectomy with tissue graft sealing.
2. Stapedotomy can be performed regularly, even in presence of minimal rim fixation if the conventional surgical steps are reversed obtaining the desired fenestra *before* disrupting the incudo-stapedial joint and/or breaking off the stapedial arch.

3. Stapedotomy performs significantly better than stapedectomy at 4000 Hz, but the hearing results between 0.5 and 2 kHz are 5 dB less good than after stapedectomy.

The statistical analysis of the results has been carried out at the Biomedical Statistical Institute of the University of Zurich (according to the Wilcoxon test by Dr. H. Helfenstein).

References

1. Marquet, J., Creten, W.L., and Van Camp, K.J. Consideration about the surgical approach in stapedectomy. *Acta Otolaryngol (Stockh)* 74: 406–410, 1972.
2. Smyth, G.D.L., and Hassard, T.H. Eighteen years experience in stapedectomy, the case of the small fenestra operation. *Ann. Otol, Rhinol, Otolaryngol* (Suppl). 49: 87, 1978.
3. Fisch, U. *Tympanoplasty and Stapedectomy.* Thieme-Stratton Inc., New York, 1980.

CHAPTER 12
Experiences with Revision Stapedectomy

James L. Sheehy, M.D.

There are many interrelated factors involved in making a decision in regard to advising a revision stapedectomy: the degree of conductive deficit, the presence of a balance disturbance or surgically related sensorineural hearing impairment, the type of otosclerotic focus, and the experience of the surgeon.

In this paper, I will make some comments on primary stapedectomy and review the results of revision stapedectomy at the Otologic Medical Group (OMG), making recommendations in regard to these interrelated factors.

PRIMARY STAPEDECTOMY

There are many techniques of stapedectomy, and almost all otological surgeons are in agreement on certain points: The prosthesis should be securely attached to the incus (or, at times, the malleus), 90% or more of the patients should have a postoperative conductive deficit of 10 dB or less and less than 1% should suffer a severe sensorineural impairment.

But there are still many controversial areas. What is the best prosthesis? Must the window opening be covered with a tissue graft? Who should perform the surgery?

At OMG, we believe that the type of prosthesis is a personal matter and probably is not a key factor, in itself, in the results of surgery. But the prosthesis must be securely attached to the incus (or malleus). We may use one of three prostheses: prefabricated wire loop (House prosthesis) (1); prefabricated wire loop-Gelfoam prosthesis for use with tissue grafts (Sheehy prosthesis) (2); and various sized pistons when the small fenestra technique is used.

For many years, we used Gelfoam over the open window. I stopped using this procedure in 1968 (3) and none at OMG have used Gelfoam as the window covering since late 1977. The incidence of sensorineural impairment, fistula, and dizziness was greater than when tissue was used over the window (4). Tissue grafts (fascia, perichondrium, or fat) were used routinely until recently when the small fenestra piston technique without a tissue covering was used by some of my associates.

Who should do the surgery? Only those individuals who have done 100 or more stapedectomies? But how is that individual to gain this experience? Only those who limit their practice to otology? Only those who have taken a postresidency otological Fellowship? Or should everyone who finishes an otolaryngology residency perform stapedectomy?

These questions are very difficult to answer. In fact, there is no answer. The number of operations performed by the individual is probably nowhere near as important as his technical ability in otological surgery and his judgment, both in selection of the patient and at the time of surgery. The problem is that there are fewer stapedectomy cases available for resident training and it is difficult to obtain this judgment and experience.

It is even more difficult to gain judgment and experience when it comes to revision of stapedectomy failures. These operations are more complicated, require more judgment (preoperatively and at surgery), and yield less satisfactory results. The remainder of this paper is limited to a discussion of revision of stapedectomy failures.

THE STUDY

The charts on 288 revision stapedectomies performed during an 8-year period were reviewed. Revisions of our own cases accounted for 80%. The 288 operations represent 8.6% of the otosclerosis surgery during the 8 years (5). Of all of the operations, 20% were performed by the author.

A variety of techniques were used in the 220 cases in which the primary surgery was performed at OMG (Table 12.1). Of the seven procedures listed only the tissue graft techniques are still used. One-third of the patients were operated on within a year of their primary surgery. One-half, however, were operated on 6 or more years later and 8% were operated on 16 years or more later.

CAUSES OF FAILURE

The cause of failure (C of F) was recorded in the record of 96% of the cases (Table 12.2). In 15%, there was more than one problem. In these cases, we recorded all problems (occurrence) and selected the one which we believed was the major factor (primary C of F).

The C of F must be interpreted in light of the technique used at the primary surgery, some of the techniques have not been used for many years or have been used only occasionally (Table 12.1). The most common primary procedure used for years was the wire-Gelfoam-pad technique (1) and this was also the single most common revision technique inasmuch as 58% of the

Table 12.1
Technique of Primary Surgery in First Revision of Cases Initially Operated on at OMG

Primary Surgery	Incidence
Footplate Fragmentation	
Polyethylene tube	7%
Wire from incus	15%
Gelfoam Membrane	
Polyethylene tube	4%
Wire from incus	57%
Wire from malleus	4%
Tissue Graft	
Wire from incus	8%
Wire from malleus	5%

Table 12.2
Causes of Failure in 288 Cases

Causes of Failure in Revision Stapedectomy	Occurrence (%)	Primary Causes of Failure (%)
Displaced prosthesis	46	41
Incus necrosis	17	5
Fistula	16	9
Short prosthesis	12	9
Bony closure	9	9
Fixed footplate	9	8
Adhesions	5	3
Fixed malleus	2	2

revisions were performed by Dr. Howard House. The Cs of F (and the results of the revision surgery) had been influenced significantly by this abandoned Gelfoam-pad procedure.

Displaced Prosthesis

Prosthesis displacement, usually to the inferior edge of the window, was the single most common C of F (41%). This was the primary C of F in two-thirds of the wire-Gelfoam procedures, one-third of which also had a fistula.

Incus Necrosis

Incus necrosis was a common C of F in the polyethylene tube (PET) prosthesis era (6) and was present in one-third of 15 such cases in this study. It was the primary C of F in only eight cases in which a PET had not been used at the primary surgery.

Oval Window Fistula

An oval window fistula was detected in 41 patients; seven of these were in the PET cases. Of the Gelfoam revisions, 20% had a fistula. None were noted in the 11 revisions in which a tissue graft had been used at the primary surgery.

Short Prosthesis

A short prosthesis was the C of F in 9%. This was the single most C of F in bluish footplate fragmentation cases (7).

Bony Closure

Bony closure of the oval window was the C of F in 23 cases (9%), 17 of which had obliterative otosclerosis. We will discuss these cases later. There was a high incidence of sensorineural hearing impairment following the revision surgery.

Fixed Footplate

The fixed footplate incidence of 9% was predominately a problem in cases in which the bluish footplate fragmentation technique had been used at the primary surgery.

PREOPERATIVE DEAD EARS

There were eight ears which had a total loss of hearing prior to the revision performed to close a possible fistula. All had had Gelfoam used as the oval window covering. The two PET cases had a fistula. No specific C of F was identified in any of the wire cases. Unsteadiness was presented in 5 of the 8 patients; in 4 of the 5, the unsteadiness subsided postoperatively and in the other a translabyrinthine nerve section was performed with a successful outcome.

HEARING RESULTS

The hearing results are reported as postoperative conductive deficit rather than closure of the airbone gap. We used the best bone conduction (BC) level, whether it occurred preoperatively or 4 months or more postoperatively, and as such, there is no possibility of so-called overclosure. Table 12.3 shows the results of the most recent hearing test in cases with 4 months or more follow-up information. Less than 50% have a 10 dB gap or less. The 6%

Table 12.3
Hearing Results in Patients with 4 Months or more Follow-Up

Postoperative Conductive Deficit	All Cases (N = 239) (%)	IRP and TORP (N = 48) (%)
10 dB or less	45	53
15 dB or less	60	65
20 dB or less	71	73
Sensorineural	6	6
Dead ear	7 cases	2 cases

incidence of sensorineural hearing impairment was much higher than anticipated and I will discuss these cases later.

There are many factors involved in the outcome of revision surgery: preoperative hearing impairment, drill out of obliterative otosclerosis and the use of Gelfoam over the window. Not apparently involved in the outcome was the presence of an oval window fistula.

Preoperative Hearing Impairment

The postoperative hearing results appear to be related to the preoperative status of the hearing. In seven cases without a preoperative hearing impairment, the results were excellent. These were cases of postoperative fluctuant conductive hearing impairment or postoperative dizziness in which a fistula was suspected. In another seven cases with a pure sensorineural hearing impairment (often with some dizziness), the results were poor; three of the seven developed a further sensorineural hearing impairment and two of these were dead ears.

Obliterative Otosclerosis

There were 17 patients who had a drill out of obliterative otosclerosis with one-half or more of the oval window being opened; 7 of the 17 had not had obliterative otosclerosis at the primary surgery; a drill was used for the first time at the revision. Five of these 7 first drill outs did well; 2 developed sensorineural impairment but still have a functioning ear, without dizziness.

Eleven patients had a drill out of obliterative otosclerosis for a second or third time; 7 of the 11 developed a sensorineural hearing impairment and 4 of these 7 lost all hearing. Two of the 3 dead ears occurred in patients who had developed unsteadiness and a sensorineural impairment after the first drill out. They were re-explored for a fistula (not found) and the surgeon decided to reopen the vestibule.

Gelfoam Cases

We were interested in determining to what extent the use of Gelfoam as an oval window covering at the revision surgery contributed to the mediocre hearing results. To do this, we compared the results of Gelfoam and tissue grafts in 105 first revisions with 4 months or more follow-up in which a drill was not used at the revision surgery. There were 33 cases in which a tissue graft was used as the revision window covering; 70% were within 10 dB and there were no sensorineural impairments. In the 72 cases in which Gelfoam was used at the revision, only 50% had a satisfactory result and six cases (8%) developed a sensorineural impairment, 1 of which was a dead ear. It appears that Gelfoam as a window covering contributed significantly to the adverse results.

Miscellaneous Comments

The results of revisions of cases initially operated on elsewhere were better than revisions of our own cases. Three-fourths of 32 first revisions were within 10 dB and there were no sensorineural impairments. The results were better in these cases initially operated elsewhere because the C of F of the primary surgery was related more to surgical technique than to oval window healing problems.

There were no differences in the hearing results when comparing the 41 fistula cases and the 247 cases without a detectable oval window fistula.

The percentage of successful hearing results was the same in the 52 patients with a balance disturbance preoperatively as it was in those cases without vestibular symptoms. Sensorineural hearing impairment following revision surgery, however, was twice as common in patients with a balance disturbance prior to the revision.

INCUS BYPASS PROCEDURES

A wire from the malleus (incus replacement prosthesis-IRP) (8) was the procedure in 43 cases. In two-thirds of these, the oval window was covered with Gelfoam, the technique preferred by Dr. Howard House at the time. Fat from the lobule of the ear (preferred by the author) (9) was used as a window covering in the other third. In 13 cases, the bypass technique was a TORP (10) to perichondrium over the window with cartilage interposed between the platform and the tympanic membrane.

Indications

Fifty percent of the bypass procedures were indicated because of incus necrosis. Other incus problems (short, fixed, dislocated) accounted for an additional 30%. Most of the remainder were cases of idiopathic malleus head fixation, the single most common indication for a bypass in primary stapedectomy (9).

Hearing Results

The residual conductive deficits following use of an IRP or TORP in revision stapedectomy are shown in Table 12.3: 65% were within 15 dB. Although these results are not as good as bypass results in primary stapedectomy (9), they are the same, in fact slightly better, than those in the other revision cases in which a prosthesis was used from the incus. This apparent inconsistency can be explained by the fact that the IRP and TORP were used in cases in which the C of F was a fixed malleus or an incus problem rather than a more difficult oval window problem.

SENSORINEURAL IMPAIRMENT

There were 18 revision operations (6%) which resulted in a severe sensorineural hearing impairment. One-half of these were dead ears. The other 9 had useful hearing remaining but decreases in discrimination of 30% or more or BC impairment of 30 dB or more or both of these. Eleven followed first revisions (5% incidence) and 6 followed second or third revisions (10% incidence).

Dead Ears

A functionless ear resulted from revision stapedectomy in nine cases (3%), four of which occurred following repeat drill outs of obliterative otosclerosis. Two of the other 5 occurred in patients who had developed inner ear symptoms (unsteadiness and sensorineural impairment) following the previous surgery. Only one of these had a fistula. All had Gelfoam used as a window covering at the revision.

Other Sensorineural Impairments

Five of the nine sensorineural cases (other than dead ears) developed following a drill out of obliterative otosclerosis. The remaining four were wire-Gelfoam cases, one of which had a fistula.

COMMENTS

To say that we were surprised by the findings of this study would be an understatement. We were disappointed in the overall hearing results and were shocked by the number of sensorineural hearing impairments. The results were, however, similar to findings in other reports (11, 12).

There were many factors involved in the adverse results: repeat drill outs of obliterative otosclerosis, opening of the inner ear when there was an unexplained balance disturbance, or sensorineural impairment and Gelfoam covering of the window.

Obliterative Otosclerosis

A repeat drill out of obliterative otosclerosis resulted in a severe sensorineural hearing impairment in seven of 10 cases, four of which lost all hearing. These operations were performed at a time when Dr. Howard House was evaluating the efficacy of sodium fluoride in preventing regrowth of bone in prior obliterative drill out failures. Obviously revision of prior drill outs is a potentially dangerous procedure. The patient should be advised of this and warned that if regrowth of bone is encountered the procedure may be terminated without help for hearing.

Inner Ear Symptoms

The patient who develops a balance disturbance or sensorineural hearing impairment, or both, following stapedectomy presents a dilemma for the otologist. Does the patient have a fistula? If a fistula is present, will it heal spontaneously? Will the hearing deteriorate further if the fistula is not closed immediately? How long should one wait to make a decision? We wish we had the answers to these questions, but we do not.

We usually do not recommend early revision (within 1-2 months) regardless of the patient's symptoms. If there is a persistent balance disturbance which incapacitates the patient, or there is a progressive sensorineural impairment, exploration of the middle ear may be indicated. At the revision of such a case, it is important that the surgeon understand that nothing should be done unless a fistula is identified. Opening of the oval window in a nonfistula case with vestibular symptoms was the probable cause of the sensorineural hearing impairment in three cases, two of which developed a dead ear.

Gelfoam

It is difficult to say with certainty how big a role Gelfoam played as a window covering in the adverse revision results, but we believe it was significant. In three previous studies, sensorineural hearing impairment or a fistula, or both, had been up to six times more common with Gelfoam than with tissue grafts over the window. Those who may still be using Gelfoam as a window covering should seriously consider discontinuing this procedure regardless of how satisfactory their results may have been.

Hazards of Revision Stapedectomy

There is no question that the hearing results in revision stapedectomy are less satisfactory than those in primary stapedectomy, but is revision stapedectomy a more hazardous procedure? The results could be interpreted that way. The incidence of sensorineural hearing impairment was over three times the incidence we would expect in our primary cases. The incidence of adverse results following multiple revisions was four times as high.

But is this a correct interpretation of the results? We think not. All but one of the sensorineural hearing impairments occurred either following a repeat drill out of obliterative otosclerosis or in a case in which Gelfoam was used as an oval window covering at the time of revision. Non-drill out first revisions with a tissue graft covering of the window did not lead to a sensorineural hearing impairment in any instance and the hearing results were better than when Gelfoam was used as a window covering.

GUIDELINES FOR REVISION STAPEDECTOMY

There are many interrelated factors involved in making a decision in regard to advising a revision stapedectomy: the degree of conductive deficit, the presence of a balance disturbance or surgically related sensorineural hearing impairment, the type of otosclerotic focus, and the experience of the surgeon.

Revision stapedectomy resulted in an excellent hearing result in less than 50% of the cases. As such, revision stapedectomy probably is not indicated in most cases when the conductive deficit is less than 20 dB unless the surgeon has had a great deal of experience and has reason to believe that there is a fistula or a lateral chain problem such as necrosis of the incus or malleus head fixation.

The oval window membrane should not be disturbed in a patient with a postoperative balance disturbance or postoperative sensorineural hearing impairment unless a surgeon identifies a fistula or a slipped or long prosthesis, i.e., a possible cause of the inner ear symptoms.

There is rarely an indication for a repeat drill out of obliterative otosclerosis.

Otolaryngologists who perform revision stapedectomy should be prepared to perform an incus bypass procedure. This was indicated in 20% of our cases.

References

1. House, H.P. The prefabricated wire loop-Gelfoam stapedectomy. *Arch Otolaryngol* 76: 298, 1962.
2. Sheehy, J.L. Stapedectomy wire prosthesis for use with tissue grafts. *Trans Am Acad Ophthalmol Otolaryng* 82: 108, 1976.
3. Sheehy, J.L., and Perkins, J.L. Stapedectomy: Gelfoam compared with tissue grafts. *Laryngoscope* 86: 436, 1976.
4. Sheehy, J.L., Nelson, R.A., and House, H.P. Stapes surgery at the Otologic Medical Group. *Am J Otol* 1: 22, 1979.
5. Sheehy, J.L., Nelson, R.A., and House, H.P. Revision stapedectomy: a review of 258 cases. *Laryngoscope* 91: 43, 1981.
6. Sheehy, J.L., and House, H.P. Causes of failure in stapes surgery. *Laryngoscope* 72: 10, 1962.
7. House, H.P., Linthicum, F.H., and House, J.W. Footplate fragmentation in otosclerosis surgery. *Laryngoscope* 80: 1256, 1970.
8. Sheehy, J.L., and Powers, W.H. Incus replacement prosthesis in otosclerosis surgery. *Arch Otolaryngol* 89: 393, 1969.
9. Sheehy, J.L. Stapedectomy: Incus bypass procedures. A report of 203 operations. *Laryngoscope* (in press) 1981.
10. Brackmann, D.E., and Sheehy, J.L. Tympanoplasty: TORPs and PORPs. *Laryngoscope* 89: 108, 1979.
11. Crabtree, J.A., Britton, B.H., and Powers, W.H. An evaluation of revision stapes surgery. *Laryngoscope* 90: 224, 1980.
12. Feldman, B.A., and Schuknecht, H.F. Experiences with revision stapedectomy procedures. *Laryngoscope* 80: 1281, 1970.

CHAPTER 13

Variable Clinical Presentations of Acoustic Tumors

Charles M. Luetje, M.D.

Seven selected case histories from 42 patients operated consecutively between October 1976 and June 1981 for removal of acoustic tumors were reviewed which showed considerable variation in clinical presentation. Hearing loss was the most common clinical symptom in all 42 cases although pure tone and speech audiometry revealed hearing loss in only 95%. Tinnitus was present in 90% and dysequilibrium in 74%.

Auditory brain stem response (ABR) when performed accurately yielded 100% abnormality. Reduced vestibular response was present in 81% and abnormal stapedial reflexes, absence or decay in 74%. An abnormal C-T scan was present in 86% (36 cases) requiring pantopaque cisternography to make the diagnosis in the remaining cases.

These histories exemplify the composite audiological, vestibular, and radiographic studies involved in the diagnosis of acoustic tumors.

A high index of suspicion remains the clinical cornerstone in the diagnosis of acoustic tumors. Two diagnostic studies have emerged in superiority, however, almost supplanting clinical suspicion, and conventional audiometric and vestibular testing. They are third generation C-T scanning and ABR capabilities.

The third generation C-T scanner, especially with review capabilities, has almost eliminated the necessity for pantopaque cisternography. In my opinion, it is the single most important diagnostic test for acoustic tumors. ABR testing has emerged as the most accurate test in the audiometric battery. However, a word of caution is necessary regarding both of these studies. Certain pitfalls occur with first and second generation C-T scanners due primarily to lack of resolution of the internal auditory canal (IAC) (1). Secondly, patients with hearing loss may exhibit wave V and interwave latencies deceiving to the inexperienced eye.

The question then arises, where does one start the clinical evaluation and when does one stop? Are an audiogram with pure tones and speech, stapedial reflexes, IAC x-rays, and ENG adequate? Should ABR be done routinely? When should a C-T scan be obtained? Should a C-T scan be obtained after the audiogram and eliminate the other tests?

This paper attempts to shed some light on these questions by providing 7 cases of variation in the presenting symptoms and evaluation of patients in whom an acoustic tumor was suspected and surgically confirmed.

CASE MATERIAL

CASE 16: A.T. A 26-year-old female developed tinnitus in the right ear and disequilibrium. Shortly this was followed by right facial and head numbness. The symptoms appeared to be intermittent at first but in 2 months, she noticed hearing loss in the right ear, headaches, nausea, and vomiting. An audiogram done 18 months later (Fig. 13.1) revealed normal hearing but absent stapedial reflexes on the right, tone decay, and rollover. Examination revealed bilateral papilledema and decreased facial sensation on the right with lid lag on eye blink. A C-T scan was performed by her referring neurologist (Fig. 13.2). On February 6, 1980, she underwent combined translabyrinthine, retrosigmoid, transtentorial total removal of this large acoustic tumor with preservation of normal facial function.

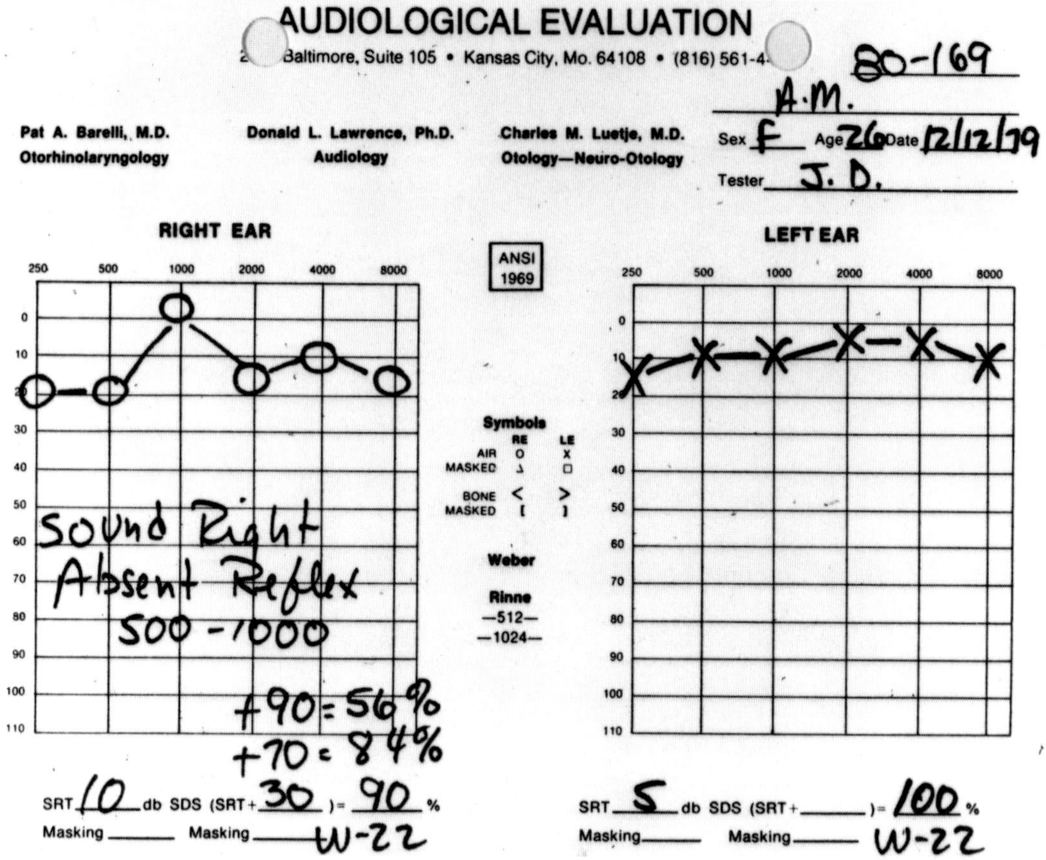

92 Clinical Otology

Figure 13.1. Audiogram, case 16, right 3.8-cm acoustic tumor.

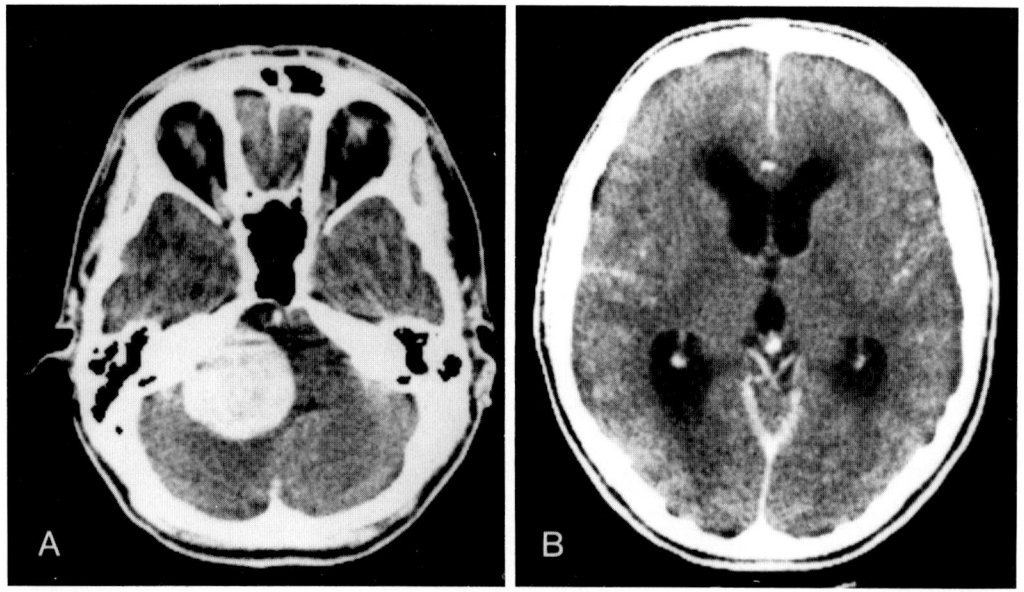

Figure 13.2. A. Large right acoustic tumor on C-T scan. B. Hydrocephalus in same patient.

Acoustic Tumors 93

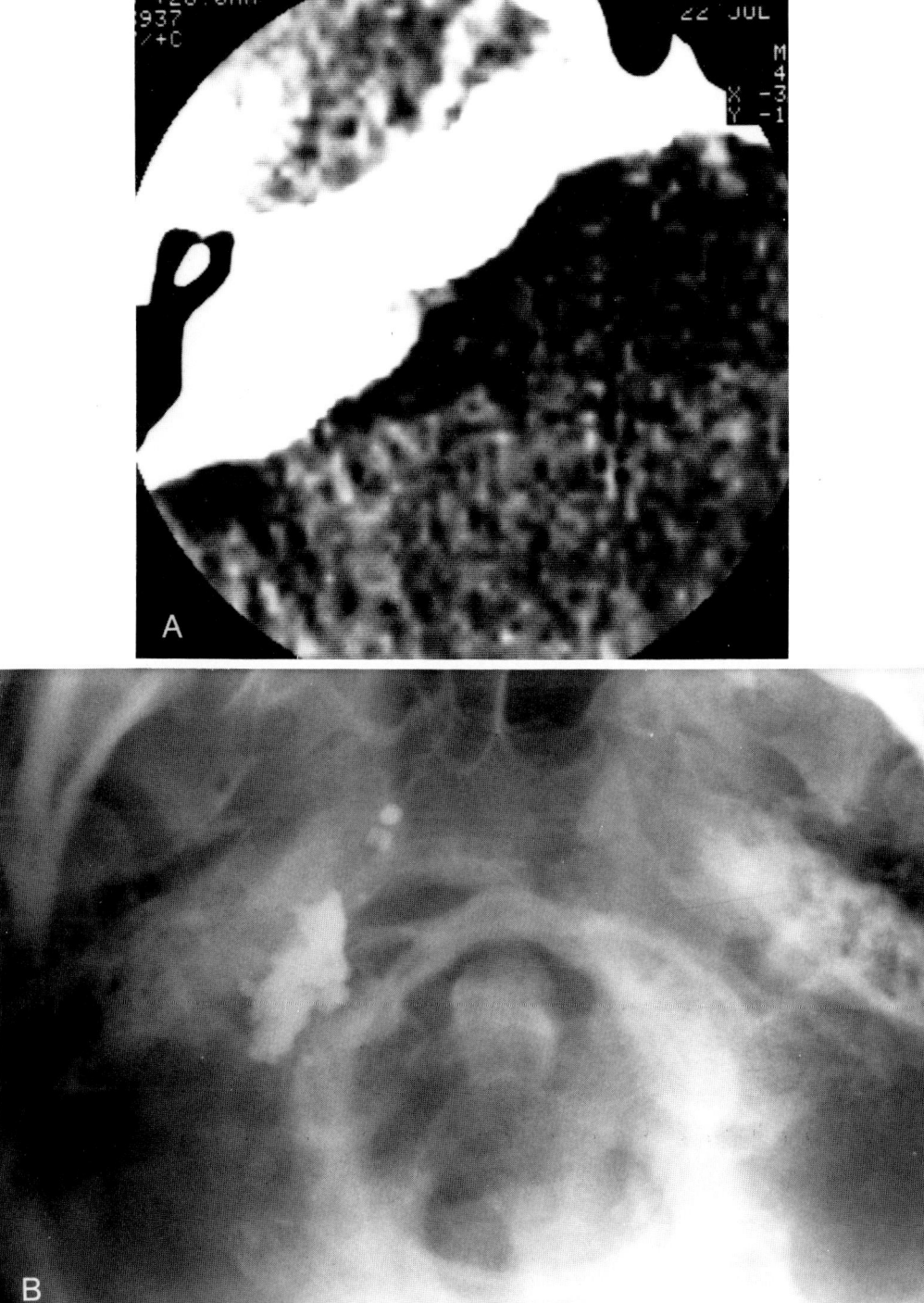

Figure 13.3. *A.* C-T scan showing predominantly intracannalicular acoustic tumor. *B.* Pantopaque in same patient outlining the tumor.

94 Clinical Otology

Comment: This patient had normal pure tone and speech audiometry but noticed subjective symptoms of hearing loss in the right ear. She presented with a very large tumor, papilledema, V and VII nerve findings, yet minimal VIII nerve findings.

CASE 25: V.S. A 52-year-old lady presented with tinnitus and unilateral sensorineural hearing loss in the right ear of 1 year's duration. Her SRT was 25 db and speech discrimination score 88% with a high tone loss. ENG showed 22% reduced vestibular response in the opposite left ear. IACs were symmetrical but the crista falciformis was poorly seen on the right and the posterior lip slightly shortened. Five months later, ABR was abnormal and the diagnosis of an acoustic tumor made on C-T scan and pantopaque cisternography (Fig. 13.3). The tumor was predominantly intracanalicular. On August 20, 1980, middle cranial fossa removal was accomplished and hearing preserved. On April 4, 1981, SRT was 40 db, speech discrimination score 80%.

Comment: Although this patient had a 25 dB SRT, 88% speech discrimination score, and high tone loss, she had no reduced vestibular function on the right and I elected to follow her for a few months. Only after an abnormal ABR did I proceed with C-T scan and pantopaque cisternography.

CASE 31: M.L. A 1.5-cm acoustic tumor was diagnosed on C-T scan in this 40-year-old female. Seven years prior to diagnosis, she had a total right facial paralysis, presumably Bell's palsy. She also noted total hearing loss in the right ear with tinnitus and severe vertigo. Symptoms improved in 2-3 weeks except hearing never seemed normal, and she had persistent tinnitus, and balance disturbance interfered with playing tennis well. Audiogram revealed a rather flat sensori-

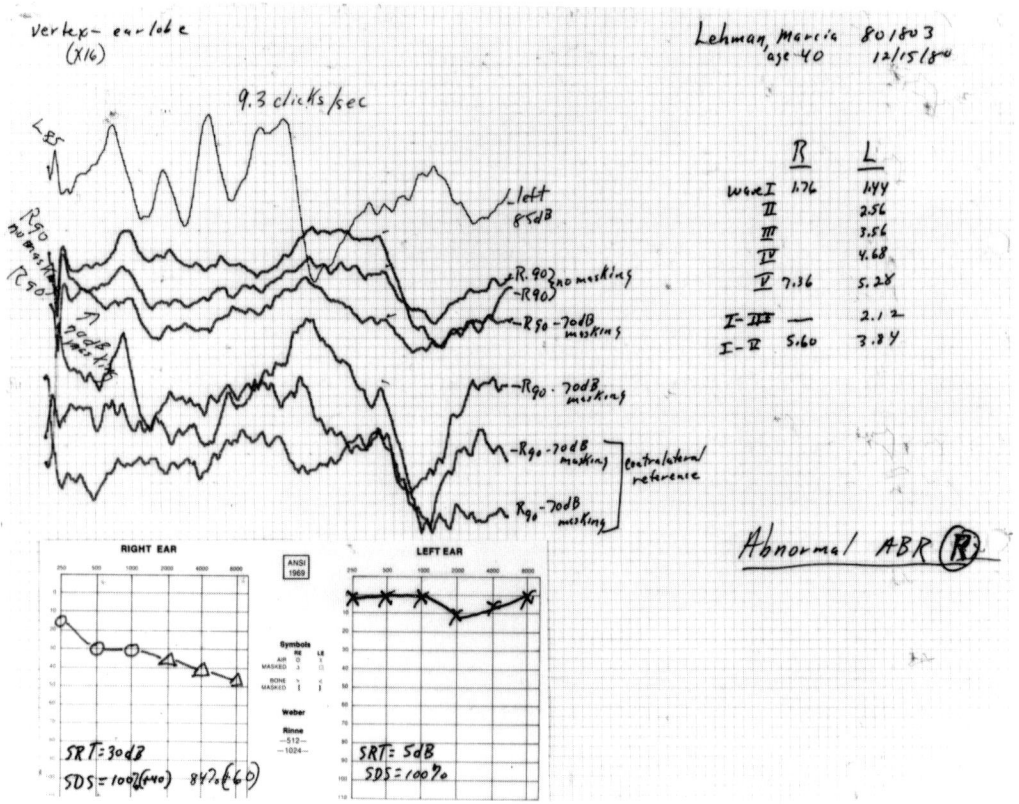

Figure 13.4. Audiogram and ABR tracing, case 31, right acoustic tumor.

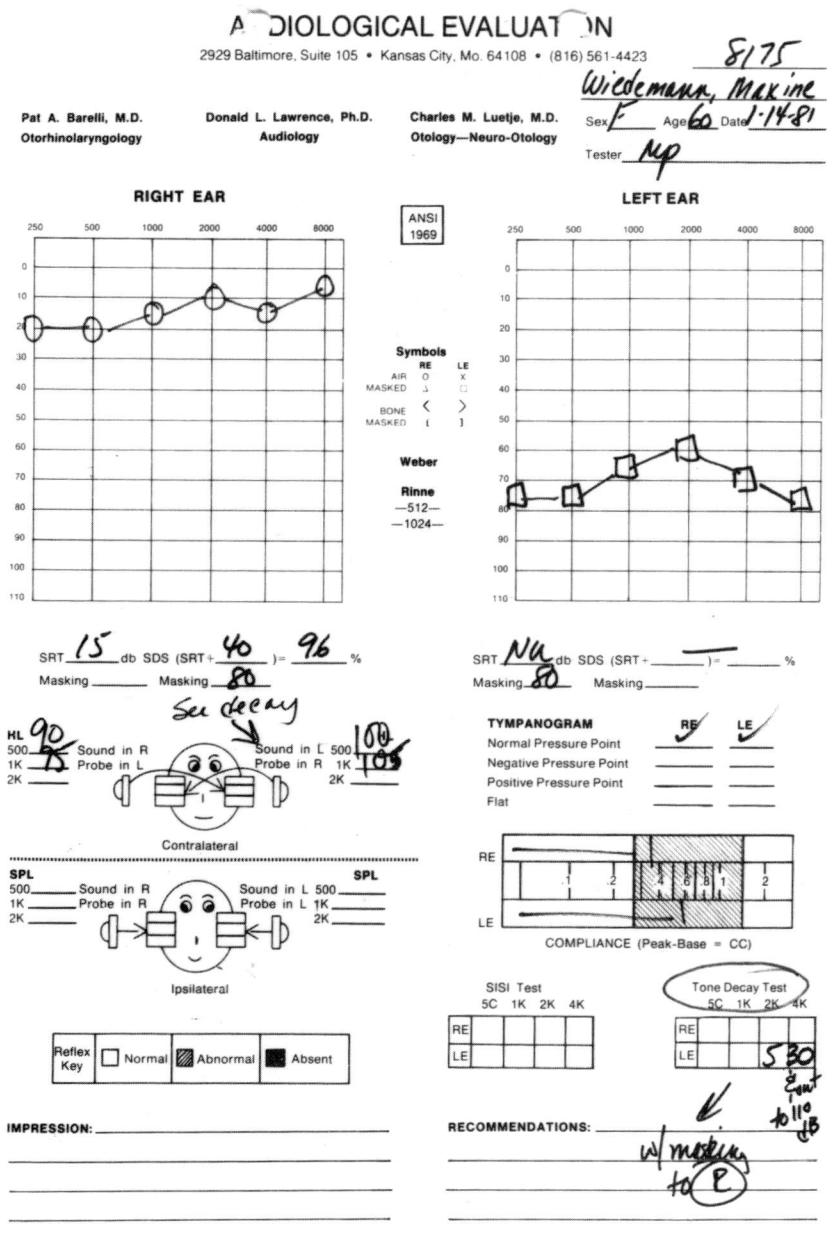

Figure 13.5. Audiogram, case 34, left acoustic tumor.

neural hearing loss at about 30 db in the right ear, 100% speech discrimination score, and an abnormal ABR (Fig. 13.4). On December 17, 1980, translabyrinthine total removal was accomplished. Facial nerve function was preserved to the level of preoperative function, with slight residual from what appeared to have been "Bell's palsy."

Comment: This patient presented 7 years prior to surgery with total right facial paralysis, no hearing, tinnitus, and severe vertigo. This was presumably Bell's palsy. However, a 1.5-cm acoustic tumor was removed 7 years later. The exact relationship between the symptoms of facial paralysis, vertigo, and hearing loss that she had 7 years ago are unknown with regards to the acoustic tumor.

CASE 34: A 60-year-old lady presented with vertigo and minimally fluctuating progressive left sensorineural hearing loss of 12 years' duration. At first, the attacks of vertigo were about a year apart and disappeared about 7–8 years ago. She had no hearing for about 5 of 6 years in the left ear. The diagnosis of Meniere's disease with vertigo, nausea, and vomiting, roaring in her left ear lasting about 4 hours. Her audiogram revealed a rather flat hearing loss with slight upsloping in the lower frequencies and no understanding for speech (Fig. 13.5). ENG showed 46% reduced vestibular response on the left especially to warm irrigation. I thought this patient had Meniere's disease and treated her medically for a month until she had her next attack "typical" of Meniere's disease. At that point, I decided to obtain a C-T scan which revealed a 1-cm acoustic tumor (Fig. 13.6). An ABR was mildly abnormal (Fig. 13.7). Total tumor removal was accomplished by translabyrinthine removal with preservation of normal VII function.

Comment: This patient had symptoms suggestive of Meniere's disease, had been diagnosed 10 years previously as Meniere's disease and, in fact, I reinitiated treatment for Meniere's disease. However, tone decay was present at 4 KHz and although her IACs appeared symmetrical, I thought there might be some shortening of the posterior lip on the left. Because of her last attack of Meniere's disease, I was considering endolymphatic sac surgery but obtained a C-T scan prior to surgery. This scan, surprisingly, showed an acoustic tumor.

CASE 30: E.H. A 66-year-old man was admitted to the hospital with acute, incapacitating vertigo and nausea. There was no history of previous balance disturbance or tinnitus. Hearing loss in the left ear was noticed 20–30 years ago and he has been unable to

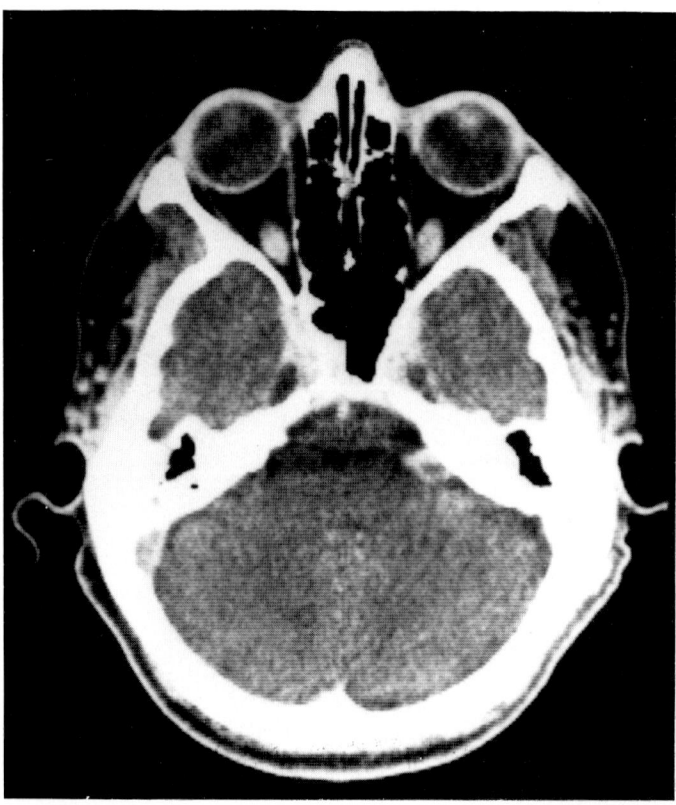

Figure 13.6 C-T scan, case 34, left acoustic tumor.

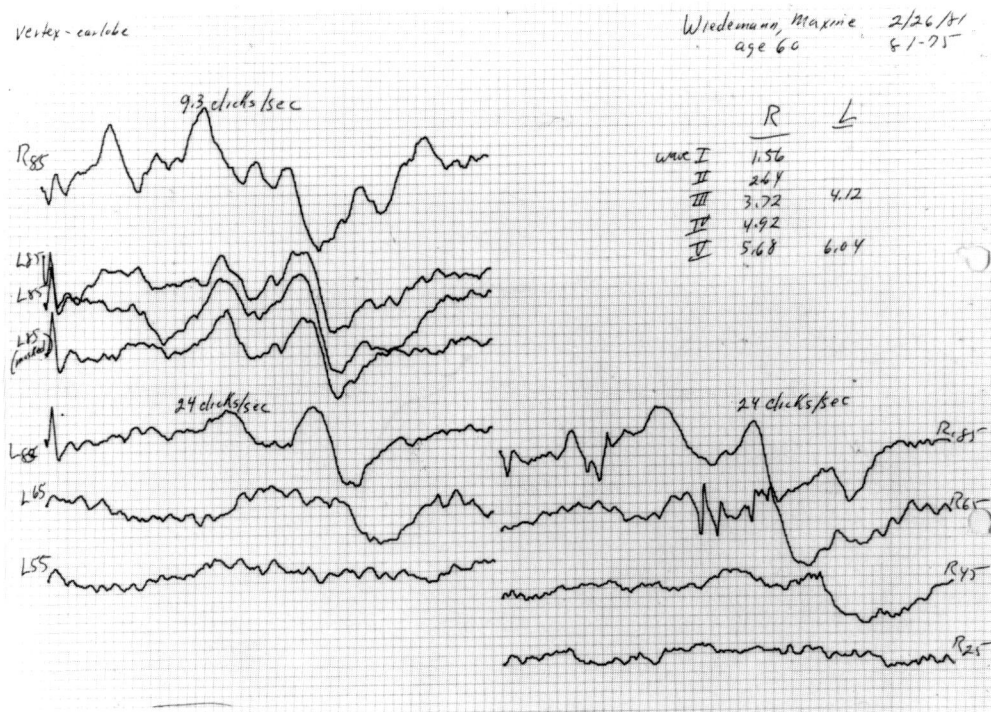

Figure 13.7. Case 34, left acoustic tumor.

hear in that ear since. A 1.5-cm left acoustic tumor was diagnosed by C-T scan. Translabyrinthine total removal was accomplished December, 1980. Hemorrhage into the center of the tumor with surrounding capsular and brain stem inflammatory reaction were present.

Comment: This patient was taking coumadin following coronary bypass surgery in 1975 and aortic valve replacement in 1980. We feel his acute vertigo was secondary to hemorrhage into the tumor and adjacent brainstem reaction. His hemorrhage could have been fatal.

CASE 39: R.W. A 23-year-old male noticed hearing loss in the right ear over the phone 1 or 2 years ago. While playing in the high school band, he noticed no hearing loss. He had no symptoms of dysequilibrium or vertigo, no tinnitus but was totally deaf in the right ear at the time of examination March 1981. C-T scan revealed a 3-cm acoustic tumor on the right. In April 1981, translabyrinthine total removal of his acoustic tumor with preservation of normal facial function was accomplished.

Comment: This is a 23-year-old individual who lost his hearing over a period of 1 or 2 years, was quite active, had no tinnitus, no disequilibrium but yet had a rather large acoustic tumor with displacement of the IV ventricle. His only complaint was hearing loss.

CASE 40: C.C. Six years ago, this 35-year-old lady had sudden onset of vertigo and slight hearing loss in the right. She noticed tinnitus for 5 or 6 years. Following acute vertigo, she has had persistent imbalance since. She had headaches for several years. Audiogram revealed normal hearing in the right ear but absent stapedial reflex and rollover (Fig. 13.8). A C-T scan was attempted during which she developed bronchospasm and the scan was aborted. IAC x-rays were normal and she had 43% reduced vestibular response to warm irrigation only. Because of the sensitivity to iodine, intrathecal pantopaque was used and did not fill the cerebellopontine

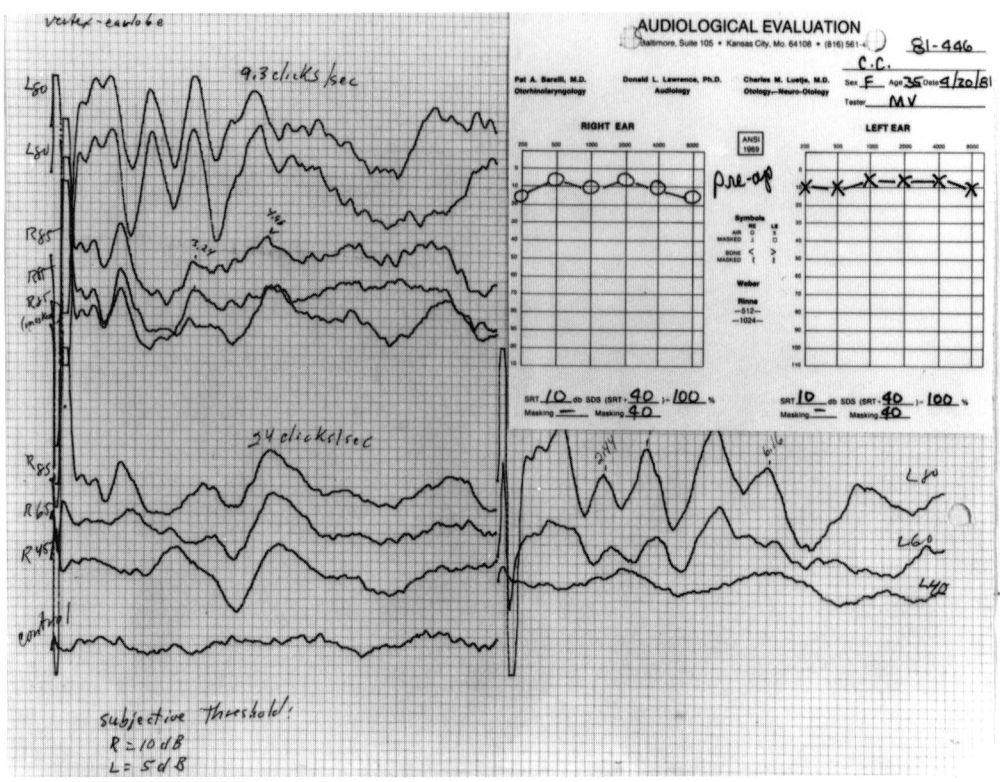

Figure 13.8. Audiogram and ABR tracing, case 40, large right acoustic tumor.

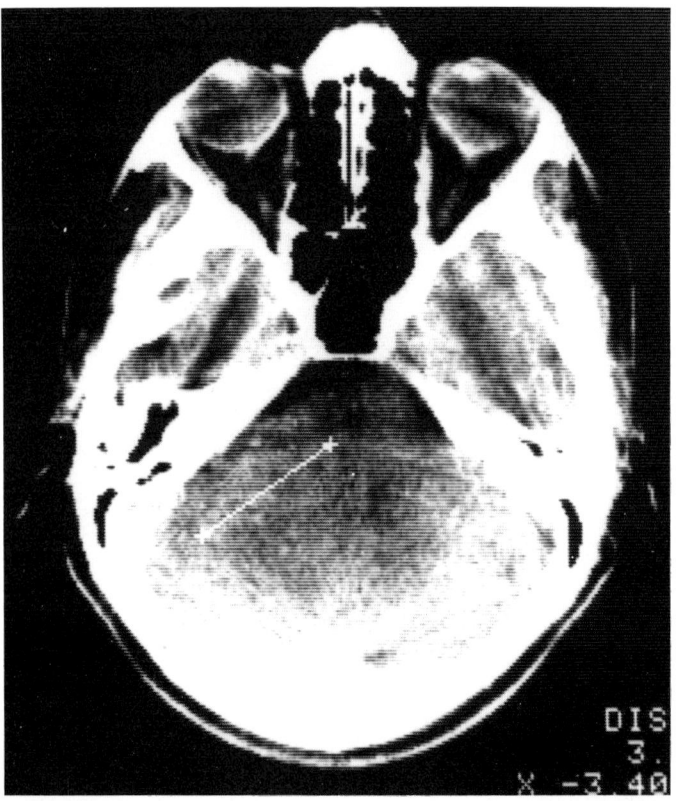

Figure 13.9 C-T scan, case 40, large right acoustic tumor.

angle. Sixteen ml of air was placed intrathecally while the patient was under the C-T scan and a 3.6-cm acoustic tumor displacing the IV ventricle was identified (Fig. 13.9). Translabyrinthine total removal was accomplished on April 22, 1981, with preservation of the facial nerve. Facial function was reduced following surgery but it is slowly recovering and we expect normal return of function.

Comment: This patient had symptoms starting with acute vertigo 6 years ago. She had normal hearing preoperatively with 100% speech discrimination score. Only the warm irrigation on ENG was reduced. She created a diagnostic problem in that she was allergic to iodine intravenously and had normal IACs. This tumor arose in the cerebellopontine angle and only after it was quite large was the diagnosis made.

DISCUSSION

Table 13.1 shows the incidence of presenting symptoms indicated by patients at their initial evaluation. Table 13.2 shows the objective findings on clinical testing. These findings are similar to those previously reported (2). A high index of suspicion is necessary for diagnosing acoustic tumors in many patients. Two of the seven patients whose case histories are reviewed were followed by the author for a few months prior to diagnosis. It is not uncommon, on the other hand, to carefully evaluate patients suspected of an acoustic tumor with all audiovestibular and x-ray studies including ABR, C-T scan, and pantopaque cisternography, only to find absence of an acoustic tumor.

Complaints of hearing loss and/or balance problems still require an orderly and complete evaluation of the audiovestibular system. If an abnormality is found with basic audiometry, ENG and LAC x-rays and a high index of clinical suspicion is present for an acoustic tumor, ABR, C-T scan and possible pantopaque cisternography are considered. Depending upon the degree of the index of suspicion, a normal ABR may stop the diagnostic process before C-T scanning. If the ABR is abnormal an enhanced C-T scan alone, with intrathecal air or C-T scan followed by pantopaque cisternography is scheduled. Because of the skill of the neuroradiologist in resolving the IAC on each side in each patient and the third generation GE scanner, the diagnostic evaluation may, in most

Table 13.1
Subjective Symptoms Prior to Diagnosis of Acoustic Tumor

Acoustic Tumors Subjective Symptoms Prior To Diagnosis (N = 42)		
	N	%
Hearing loss	42	100
Tinnitus	38	90
Disequilibrium	31	73.8
Vertigo	6	14.2
Headache	6	14.2
Ear discomfort	6	14.2
Facial numbness	5	11.9
Nausea and Vomiting	2	4.7
Fullness, pressure	1	2.3
VII weakness	1	2.3
VII paralysis	1	2.3

Table 13.2
Findings at Diagnosis of Acoustic Tumor

Acoustic Tumors Findings at Diagnosis (N = 42)		
	N	%
Hearing loss	40/42	95
Acoustic reflex		
Absence	16/39	41
Decay	9/39	23
Normal	10/39	25.6
Abnormal	4/39	10.2
Other cranial nerve involvement		
V facial numbness	10/42	23.8
VII facial weakness	2/42	4.7
Reduced vestibular response (greater than 20%)	30/37	81
Abnormal IAC films	32/36	88.9
Normal IAC films	4/36	11.1
Abnormal ABR	27/27	100
Abnormal C-T scan	36/42	85.7
Normal C-T scan*	6/42	14.3
Positive pantopaque	12/12	100

* Last negative C-T scan was February 1979 on 13th patient.

instances, stop here. Occasionally, if the scan is negative and the index of suspicion high, a pantopaque cisternogram follows the scan immediately in an adjoining x-ray room. One must see each IAC adequately demonstrated in each patient on C-T scan to assure a precise study. Older generation C-T scanners and improperly monitored third generation C-T scans may lead to false negatives.

CONCLUSION

The diagnosis of an acoustic tumor, in most instances, is a composite study of audiovestibular function and radiographic demonstration by computed enhanced tomography. The index of clinical suspicion should remain high but practical in patients with unilateral hearing loss, tinnitus, and balance disturbance. Considerable variation occurs in the clinical presentation of patients with acoustic tumors. Complacency should not occur in evaluating patients whose symptoms are similar to those in the cases presented in this paper.

References

1. Luetje, C.M. The C-T scan: Pitfalls and posterior fossa cisternography. *Otolaryngol Head Neck Surg 87:* 266–267, 1979.
2. Graham, M.D. Acoustic tumors: Selected histories and patient reviews. In: Acoustic Tumors: Diagnosis. House, W.F. and Luetje, C.M. (Eds). Vol. 1, University Park Press, Baltimore, 1979.

CHAPTER 14
Middle Cranial Fossa Surgery

Lee A. Harker, M.D.

The temporal bone contains the essentials of the sound conducting and translating mechanism, the peripheral vestibular apparatus, and the peripheral portions of the sensory nerves subserving these sense organs. Portions of the carotid artery, jugular bulb, and facial nerve are also surrounded by this complex bone. This paper presents a brief state-of-the-art of otologic middle cranial fossa surgery.

Although the neurosurgical approach to the middle cranial fossa has been practiced since Frank Hartley's description of an approach to the Gasserian ganglion in 1892 (1), the otologic frontier was not opened until August 1st, 1959, when William House operated upon his first patient. In 1961, he described 14 cases in his Triologic thesis (2) and by 1963, he published his first 50 cases (3). The introduction of modern otologic techniques into a field occupied solely by neurosurgeons was substantially a one-man endeavor, and there have been few refinements or additions to the technique that Dr. House described.

Although several different surgical procedures for various disease processes have been carried out by this approach throughout the years, the most common contemporary indications involve gaining access to the nerves traversing the temporal bone. The most frequent use is for total or partial vestibular nerve section as treatment for persistent, unilateral, peripheral vestibular dysfunction. It is possible to permanently interrupt the fluctuating barrages of ipsilateral neural impulses from a diseased labyrinth, usually preserving existing auditory function. Since the neural transection is at or central to the ganglion of Scarpa, axonal degeneration to the second order vestibular neurons occurs, and there is no opportunity for recurrence of symptoms from traumatic neuroma formation at the surgical site, as has been documented following labyrinthectomy (4).

The second common indication for the otologic middle cranial fossa approach is the removal of internal auditory canal (IAC) mass lesions. Although House successfully clipped an anterior inferior cerebellar artery aneurysm, and lipomas and other unusual tumors have been reported, IAC tumors are almost exclusively schwannomas. In the past decade, two technical advances have increased the accuracy of diagnosis and, as they become more available, will allow earlier detection of smaller tumors. Electric Response Audiometry has emerged as the single best noninvasive test and air contrast cisternography with fourth generation computerized tomographic (CT) scanning yields tumor delineation far superior to positive contrast cisternography with or without older CT scanners.

The other principal utilization of the otologic middle cranial fossa (MCF) approach is in facial nerve surgery. The intracanalicular, labyrinthine, and horizontal portions of the nerve are readily accessible by this route and there is no other reliable access to the labyrinthine segment which can preserve hearing and vestibular function. The next few years should bring some clarification in the role of surgery for the acute facial palsies; if the concepts and work of Fisch and Esslen (5) are substantiated by others, some order will emerge from the current chaos. Similar clarification is needed in the treatment of traumatic facial paralysis secondary to temporal bone fracture. There can be no argument that surgical exploration is needed after a temporal bone fracture which damages the facial nerve in the region of the geniculate ganglion, causes an immediate total paralysis with subsequent degeneration, but preserves hearing. The MCF approach is the operative avenue of choice in this situation and in many other traumatic paralyses, although indications are not always as clear.

Other infrequent surgical indications include exposure of the carotid artery for protection during temporal bone resection or for control in removal of large glomus tumors, repair of MCF cerebrospinal fluid leaks, resection of petrous apical epidermoids, biopsy of apical neoplasms, and the occasional removal of petrous apex infection.

Although the procedure is a temporal craniotomy, the general assessment of the patient is concerned more with an ability to withstand general anesthetic of 2 or more hours than with specific neurosurgical risks per se. The postoperative effects on these patients due specifically to the surgical approach are minimal, certainly much less than for an abdominal or thoracic procedure.

An accurate preoperative assessment of the function of the cranial nerves is essential since several can be at risk. Special care to document trigeminal, abducens, facial, cochlear, and vestibular function should be taken.

The most accurate assessment of the topographic anatomy of the temporal bone possible should be available to the surgeon planning and executing these operations, especially in cases with temporal bone fractures, where anatomic relations are disturbed. The best current methods are hypocycloidal polytomography and CT scanning. Such studies can determine whether the superior semicircular canal directly underlies the arcuate eminence or whether there is 1–3 mm bone between the two and if that bone contains air cells or not. The degree of pneumatization at the apex has an important effect on surgical exposure. Wider retraction and better visualization are obtained in an extensively pneumatized temporal bone; the bone is larger and the exposure of the internal auditory canal and the cerebellopontine angle is better. Some situations allow the surgeon to take certain liberties. For example, with an intracanalicular schwannoma in a large IAC of a well-pneumatized temporal bone, it is possible to initiate the bone removal for IAC exposure directly over the medial aspect of the IAC itself, without previous identification of the geniculate ganglion and labyrinthine facial nerve segment or the superior semicircular canal. In this situation, time can be saved without increased risk.

A final preoperative consideration concerns previous inflammatory conditions such as purulent meningitis. The increased bleeding and risks during elevation of the scarred, adherent dura must be weighed against the benefits of surgery.

The essence of such surgical procedures can be reduced to five steps; the temporal craniotomy, exposure of the operative area by dural and brain retraction, identification of pertinent landmarks, completion of the individual surgical procedure, and wound closure.

After a 3 inch surgical shave above and anterior to the involved ear, an indwelling Foley catheter is placed and its function checked. Forty to 50 mg of furosemide are given intravenously to effect diuresis and facilitate brain retraction. Muscle relaxant agents are not used.

Utilizing opposing skin and muscle flaps above the auricle or a linear pretragal incision, the periosteum is exposed and a 4-cm temporal craniotomy performed. The dura is elevated under direct vision and small blood vessels are electrocoagulated with the bipolar coagulator. Elevation proceeds posteriorly to the length of the superior petrosal sinus; anteriorly to the region of the middle meningeal artery and medially past the arcuate eminence, facial hiatus, and the region of the geniculate ganglion as far as possible; at which point the self-retaining dural retractor is secured. Care is taken in the region of the geniculate ganglion to observe for an exposed portion of the facial nerve. The steps of the individual procedure to be performed will vary after exposure is obtained and articles dealing with these specific operations should be consulted. Suffice it to say that extensive laboratory dissection is necessary to understand the complex structural relationships within the temporal bone as viewed from this approach.

After completion of the procedure, the goals of closure should include the preservation of sterility, avoidance of damage to any exposed intratemporal structures, and the prevention of any leakage of cerebrospinal fluid into the temporal bone air cell system or from the wound. To help accomplish these goals, we copiously irrigate the wound periodically throughout the case, and utilize intra- and postoperative antibiotics for 24 hours. A small, tightly rolled, compressed Gelfoam pad is placed within a disc of temporalis fascia and very gently wedged into the surgical defect created in the IAC so that the fascia seals the dural incision and the Gelfoam expands to seal the fascia against the bone edges. Exposed apical air cells are sealed with bone wax.

Narcotics are avoided during the first 24 hours. The head of the bed is elevated 20–30° and fluid intake restricted to 1200 ml/day for 5 days to discourage cerebrospinal fluid leakage. The patients usually leave the hospital between the 5th and 10th postoperative days.

It is not possible to assess separately those complications due entirely to the surgical exposure and those which might result from the individual operation performed through that exposure. However, the access itself carries certain risks including vascular complications, cerebrospinal fluid leakage, meningitis, and brain damage, all of which are potentially life-threatening. Specific procedures may increase the possibility of some of these and may also put the patient at risk for functional deficits such as hearing loss, dysequilibrium, and facial paralysis.

Review of several published series of otologic MCF operations totaling more than 600 patients (6–14) revealed some interesting statistics. There were but 2 deaths reported, and 2 serious vascular complications, 1 of which occurred 24 hours postoperatively and was responsible for 1 of the deaths. The second was a subdural hematoma recognized and treated appropriately at the time of the original surgery. Three cases of meningitis were mentioned and 6 cases of cerebrospinal fluid leakage. No case of increased neurologic deficit indicative of brain damage was mentioned in these reviews.

Although it may be possible that some serious complications were inadvertently omitted, the complication points out the general safety of this surgical approach in the hands of experienced, skilled surgeons. A surgical mortality of 0.33% is acceptable for any craniotomy and an incidence of 1% for the most frequent serious complication is similarly tolerable. In fact, these articles document a remarkable safety record and a near freedom from serious complications despite the fact that the procedures are recognized uniformly as difficult.

Because of the inherent difficulties, it can be concluded that these procedures are best performed by surgeons with considerable experience in both laboratory dissection and otologic surgery. Also, in the United States, neurosurgical availability is a requirement since the potential operative complications may exceed the limits of otoneurosurgical training. Additionally, the published series deal almost exclusively with adult patients; it cannot be assumed that the approach is equally safe in children.

Perhaps because of these considerations, there often appears to be a certain reluctance on the part of otolaryngologists to refer patients for consultation when MCF surgery is a therapeutic alternative. We feel this is unwarranted since the procedures, by and large, are safe, effective, and often necessary for optimum patient care.

References

1. Hartley, F. Intercranial neurectomy of the second and third divisions of the Vth nerve: A new method. *New York Med J* 55: 317–319, 1892.
2. House, W.F. Surgical exposure of the internal auditory canal and its contents through the middle cranial fossa. *Laryngoscope* 71: 1363–1385, 1961.
3. House, W.F. Middle cranial fossa approach to the petrous pyramid: A report of 50 cases. *Arch Otolaryngol* 78: 406–469, 1963.
4. Linthicum, F.H., Jr., Alonso, A., and Denia, A. Traumatic neuroma: A complication of tran-

scanal labyrinthectomy. *Arch Otolaryngol* 105: 654-655, 1979.
5. Esslen, E. *The Acute Facial Palsies.* Springer-Verlag, Berlin, 1977.
6. Portmann, M., Bebear, J.P., and Lacaze, J.L. Neurectomie de la VII paire cranienne par voie de la fosse cerebrale moyenne. *Cahiers ORL* 7: 787-793, 1972.
7. Gavilan, C., and Sarria, M.J. La seccion del nervio vestibular como tratamiento sintomatico del hidrops endolinfatico. *Acta ORL* 23: 90-111, 1972.
8. Sterkers, J.M., Jobert, F., Nicolas-Charles, P., et al. Neurectomie vestibulaire et equilibre. *Probl Actuels Otorhinolaryngol* 23: 89-113, 1973.
9. Glasscock, M.F. Vestibular nerve section. *Arch Otolaryngol* 97: 112-114, 1973.
10. Smyth, G.D.I., Kerr, A.G., and Gordon, D.S. Vestibular nerve section for Meniere's disease. *J Laryngol Otolaryngol* 80: 823-831, 1976.
11. Fisch, U.: Surgical treatment of vertigo. *J Laryngol Otolaryngol* 90: 75-86, 1976.
12. Harker, L.A., and McCabe, B.F. Iowa results of acoustic neuroma operations. *Laryngoscope* 88: 1904-1911, 1978.
13. Palva, T. Vestibular neurectomy. *Acta Otolaryngol* (Suppl). 360: 51-53, 1979.
14. Garcia-Ibanez, J.L., Garcia-Ibanez, E., and Beltran de Scals, J. Hearing results after vestibular neurectomy. *Audiology* 18: 145-156, 1979.

# CHAPTER 15

Auditory Brainstem Response (Short Latency)

Earl R. Harford, Ph.D.

It has been nearly 20 years since brain stem auditory evoked potentials showed signs of becoming a useful and practical clinical procedure, mainly because of the application of the average response computer. Today, auditory brain stem response audiometry is considered a valid index of the capacity of the human ear to transmit acoustic information to the brain.

Early reports of human auditory brain stem response could only speculate on the actual nature of what was being measured. Thus, there was some disagreement on what to call the response. Nomenclature varied concerning these stable events recorded easily with noninvasive surface electrodes. For example, we find in the literature a variety of terms, such as surface-recorded responses, far-field electrocochleography, electric response audiometry, cochlear audiometry, brain stem electric response audiometry, brain stem evoked potentials, brain stem auditory responses, evoked potential audiometry, auditory pathway electric responses, brain stem evoked response audiometry, surface recorded electrocochleography, auditory evoked response audiometry, auditory brain stem response audiometry, and several others. This array of terminology added more confusion to the volumenous literature emerging on this subject, starting in the late 1960's. Finally, the joint USA-Japan Seminar on Auditory Responses from the Brain Stem, held in January 1979, unanimously recommended adoption of the term Auditory Brainstem Response, or ABR (1). In the past 2 years use of the term ABR has gained rapid popularity throughout the literature.

A principle motive for the development of ABR was to provide a clinical technique for assessing the integrity of a young child's peripheral auditory mechanism. The goal was to make audiometry as automatic and objective as possible in order to assess the auditory sensitivity of babies and difficult-to-test children. By 1967, electrocochleography was being used to record the cochlear microphonic, the summating potential, and the action potential of the eighth nerve in the human ear. The best recordings were obtained when a needle electrode was passed through the tympanic membrane to make contact with the promontory. Less invasive electrode placements in the ear canal were also used, but with much less success. Electrocochleography or ECochG was adopted enthusiastically by some otologists, but it has now been largely displaced by ABR which is much less invasive. Early commercial instrumentation for electric response audiometry was designed for slow or late cortical responses and failed to meet the need for young children and difficult-to-test patients who require sedation, which precludes accurate interpretation of cortical responses. But, by the mid-1970's, commercial instruments began to appear on the market that allowed for the recording of early potentials' i.e., within the first 10 msec following the introduction of a stimulus to the ear. These recordings are made from electrodes placed on the scalp and ear lobes, unaffected by sedation or sleep, and give as much information about the status of the cochlea as ECochG. Furthermore, these recordings give information about the status of the auditory pathway to the brain which ECochG does not provide (2).

STIMULI

ABR stimuli are characterized by abrupt onset and decay, and short duration, unlike the sustained pure tones of conventional audiometry. These stimulus parameters are necessitated by the very rapid response of the cochlea to acoustic stimulation and by the diagnostic significance of response differences of less than a millisecond. Two general types of stimulus are employed:

1. The *click* stimulus, which is by far the most popular, consists of a brief, single-polarity pulse. Its energy spectrum is composed of a broad series of harmonies of the stimulus repetition frequency, limited in the high frequency region (i.e., 1–4 kHz) by the characteristics of the earphone response and its amplifier. The click is most useful in the assessment of the auditory system where frequency-specific information is not required.

2. The second type of stimulus is the tone pip or more technically the *logon*, which is typically a 1.5-cycle burst of the desired stimulus frequency, with onset and decay times equal to 0.75 cycles of that frequency. Its waveform is a single major peak, preceded and followed by minor peaks of opposite polarity. The band width of the logon's energy spectrum is about one octave. The stimulus is more frequency specific than the click and has potential to provide a more detailed exploration of the auditory system for frequencies from 0.5–4 kHz. To date, however, the clinical efficacy of tone pips lacks adequate documentation. Currently, the most popular ABR stimulus is the click.

Auditory evoked brainstem responses are very small; i.e., about 1 microvolt in amplitude. This voltage is usually measured at the vertex or high forehead with respect to the ipsilateral ear lobe or surface of the mastoid process of the temporal bone. Actually, the intracranial voltages are much greater than a microvolt, but the intervening bone and tissue attenuate these several orders of magnitude at the skin surface.

Jewett et al. (3) and Sohmer and Feinmesser (4) were among the first to report brainstem responses from humans that seemed unaffected by sedation, sleep, or state of awareness. A year later, Jewett and Williston (5) published their classic paper describing ABR properties in humans. They demonstrated that the normal human ABR consists of 5–7 vertex positive waves occuring in the first 9 msec following a click stimulus (Fig. 15.1). This series of waves is now often referred to as "Jewett bumps."

Almost the instant of a peak stimulus impact in the tympanic membrane, a wave is induced in the fluid of the cochlea. The first indication of electrical activity generated in the hair cells is recorded about 1.6 msec following the stimulus peak. This is Jewett's Wave I which has an average amplitude of 0.15 microvolts (11). About 4 msec later, this stimulus reaches the region of the mid-brain and initiates a massive neural discharge manifest as Wave V or the IV–V complex, as it is often called in the U.S., excluding St. Louis, where it is called P_6. In Europe, it is referred to as "Sohmer 4." This robust component wave has an average amplitude of 0.38 microvolts (11).

ANATOMICAL ORIGINS

From the earliest days of ABR, there has been speculation about the anatomical origin of the component waves. There is little doubt that Wave I reflects activity of the

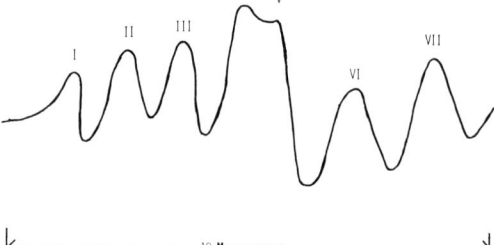

Figure 15.1. Illustration of typical ABR elicited by high intensity clicks in normal adult subjects. The response consists of seven waves occuring within the first 9 msec following the introduction of the clicks. The waves are designated by Roman numerals. Typically, positive waves at the vertex are displayed as compressions in the wave form.

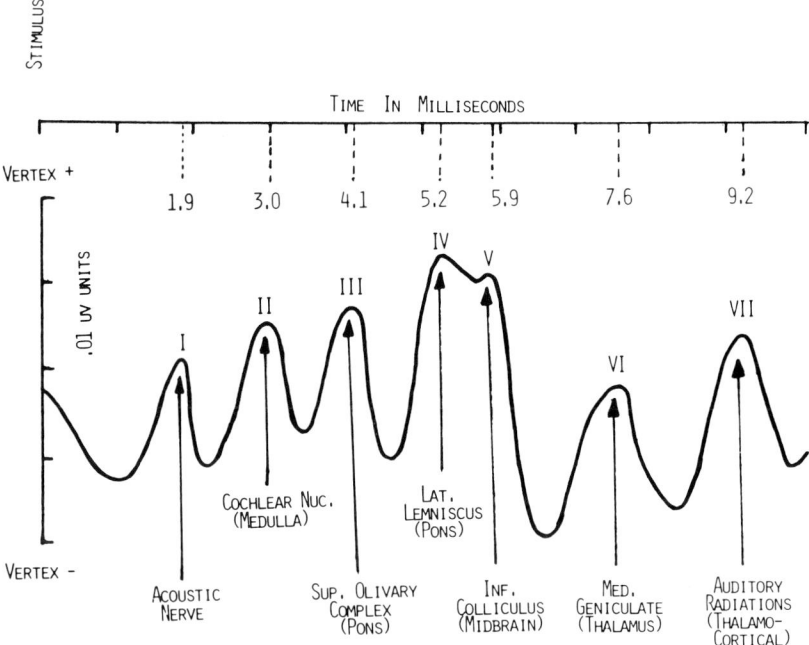

Figure 15.2. Schematic of the presumed relation between ABR component Waves and anatomical structures in the ascending auditory pathway.

bipolar cells of the eighth cranial nerve. The actual anatomical origin of the succeeding waves II–VII is mainly speculation. For the time being, the origins cited in Figure 15.2 are often used as guide posts for the seven waves that appear in the first 10 msec in the health mature auditory system.

RESPONSE PARAMETERS

In order to interpret auditory evoked potentials for clinical purposes, one must be cognizant of normal ABR characteristics and factors that can influence these features. There are three major ABR parameters; 1) morphology of the wave form, 2) absolute, interaural, and interwave latencies, and 3) absolute and relative amplitude of the waves. Variations from normal characteristics can result from changes in procedure and stimuli as well as pathological conditions. Those using ABR must obtain recordings on a group of normal subjects and maintain their normative data for clinical interpretation. Furthermore, it is important to adopt consistent stimulus parameters and procedural protocol for clinical application, which helps simplify interpretation of test results.

Morphology refers to the subjective appearance, shape, or quality of the waveform. Waveform morphology is not a quantifiable parameter. For example, Figure 15.3 shows two waveforms from the same patient, one from the right ear and one from the left ear. The left is normal, but the right manifests gross morphological degragation. Both Rowe (6) and Chiappa et al. (7) have reported investigations on normal adults that show some difference in morphology between ears in up to 20% of their study groups. The differences were rather small, but they do exist in some cases.

Absolute wave latency refers to the time between the introduction of a stimulus to the ear and elicitation of a response. Interwave latency is the interval between specified component waves (Fig. 15.4). These latencies are specified in milliseconds. Table 15.1 summarizes absolute latency for Waves 1–V from four published reports.

108 Clinical Otology

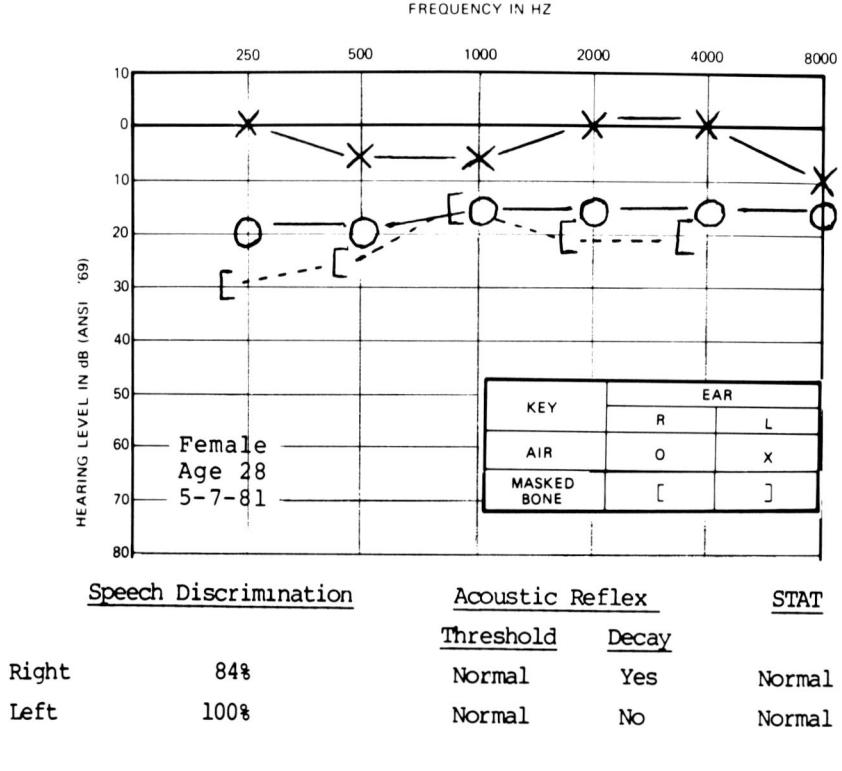

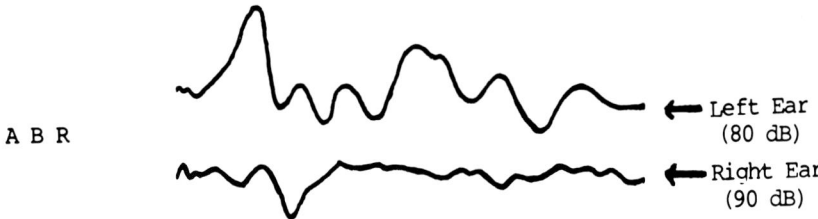

Figure 15.3. Audiogram ABR recordings for a patient with essentially normal hearing sensitivity who reports a 10-month history of lightheadedness, dizziness, and tinnitus in the left ear. The evoked responses for the right ear are normal while the left ear shows marked degradation in morphology.

Notice that the absolute wave latency of ABR component waves, when elicited by fairly loud clicks, is approximated by the Roman numeral designating the wave; i.e., Wave I occurs between 1–2 msec, Wave II between 2–3 msec, etc. The majority of reports, and especially those within the past 6 years, cite the same standard deviation for normal latency values of 0.3 msec or less. Interaural latency differences normally range between 0.2 to 0.4 msec. These standard deviations must be taken into account when interpreting interaural latency differences.

Table 15.2 displays reported data for the popular interwave latencies. The I–III interwave latency presumably specifies the transmission time of the click through the pontomedullary junction and lower pons. The III–V values represent transmission time from caudal pons to caudal midbrain levels. The I–V latency approximates the time for electrical impulses to travel the entire system, which is sometimes referred to as central conduction time or "brain stem transmission time" (8).

Two features of the amplitude of the ABR component wave have received some attention in the literature. Absolute amplitude is the number of microvolts (uv) from the peak of the wave to the following trough. The absolute amplitude can also be expressed in relation to one another which are called relative amplitude (see Fig. 15.5).

There are substantial variations of normal values for ABR wave amplitudes reported in the literature (7, 9, 10, 11). Consequently, the absolute or relative amplitude of the ABR wave is not yet commonly used in clinical practice, unless there is an obvious unmistakeable difference between a patient's two ears.

CLINICAL APPLICATIONS

Recall that the impetus for the development of ABR as a clinical procedure was to assess the auditory sensitivity of babies and young difficult-to-test children. Indeed, this goal is being met with enthusiastic success today and refinements in its application will continue to emerge from further research. One of the most significant contributions is the application of ABR to the early identification of peripheral hearing disorders in neonates. For example, here at the University of Minnesota Hospitals, we use a CRIB-O-GRAM, a microprocessor screening instrument, in our Neonatal Intensive Care Unit. All the babies in this Unit are at high risk for deafness. From the experiences reported by others, we expect to find that

Table 15.1
Normal Adult Mean Absolute Latency for ABR Component Waves I–V as Derived from a Composite of Four Published Reports (N = 145) using Similar Stimulus Parameters (6, 7, 10, 11)

Wave Component	I	II	III	IV	V
Absolute latency (msec)	1.75	2.85	3.85	5.05	5.65

Click Intensity = 60–65 dB; Filter = 100–3000 Hz

Table 15.2
Typical Interwave Latency Values Derived from Table 15.1

Interwave	I–III	III–V	I–V
Latency (msec)	1.10	1.80	3.90

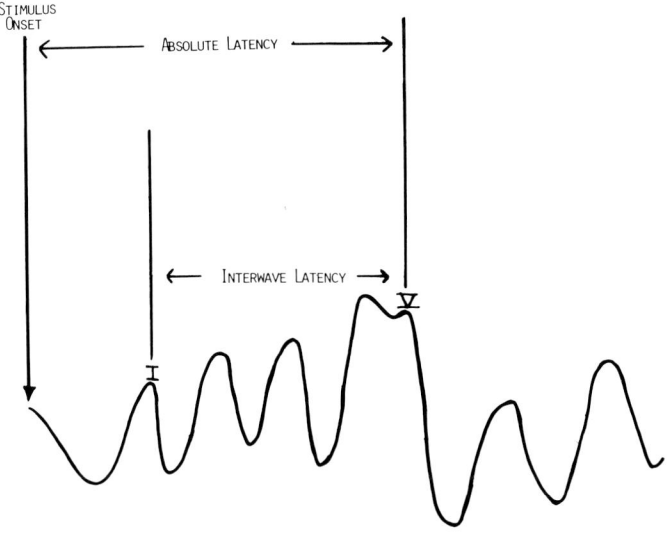

Figure 15.4 The distinction between absolute and interwave latency for component waves of the ABR. Absolute latency is the time (in msec) from the onset of a stimulus to the formation of a specific Wave peak. Interwave latency is the difference between the absolute latencies of two ABR waves.

10% of those babies who survive have a significant hearing loss (2). All those who fail the CRIB-OGRAM are seen for ABR and will be followed in the months ahead to validate the results of the ABR.

The greatest impact ABR has had on our clinical practice is for children in the age range 6-24 months and older multiply-handicapped youngsters. In years gone by, these are the children who had to make frequent trips to the audiologist for repeat testing to verify clinical speculation and hunches about the status of their hearing. In our case, many of these children are referred from hundreds of miles away. Their local health care facilities are adequate for the major portion of their clinical population, but they do not have the demand to justify expensive technical talent and instruments for special problems. Thus, they look to centers like ours for help with these complex problems. Now, when traditional behavioral audiometry cannot be used or leaves us in doubt about the status of a child's auditory sensitivity, we turn to ABR. Ordinarily, we are able to obtain definitive information and send the parents and child home the same day.

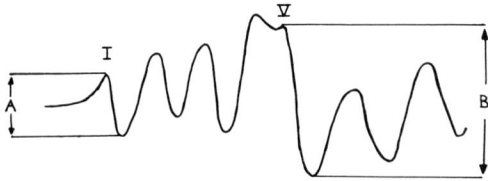

Figure 15.5. Example of wave amplitude for an ABR recording. Absolute wave amplitude is the height (in microvolts) of the wave from its peak to the following trough (A and B). Relative amplitude is the ratio of the absolute amplitude of two Waves. In this example, the relative amplitude Wave V to Wave I is $\frac{B}{A}$.

Figures 15.6 and 15.7 illustrate examples of ABR results we obtained on a newborn and a young difficult-to-test child, respectively. In brief, we have found that ABR audiometry provides an invaluable cross-check on behavioral and impedance audi-

4 Day Old ♂ Goldenhar's Syndrome
Date: 7/6/81

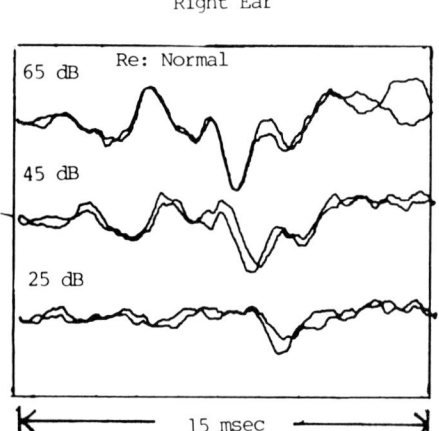

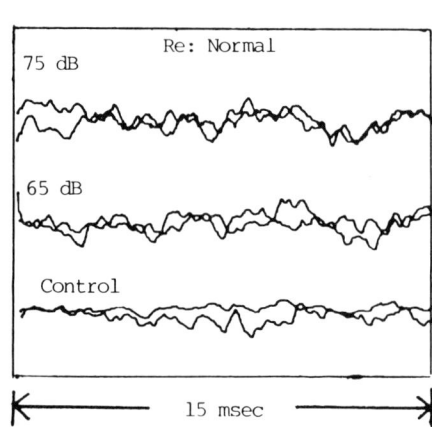

Figure 15.6. ABR results for a 4-day-old full-term newborn patient with a diagnosis of Goldenhar's syndrome with multiple anomalies, including bilateral preauricular skin tags with a great number on the right and a right hypoplastic mandible. There is also a tissue defect at the right corner of the mouth. ABR verifies essentially normal auditory sensitivity for the left ear, but a significant loss for the right ear. ABR for bone conduction stimulation will be done at 6 months.

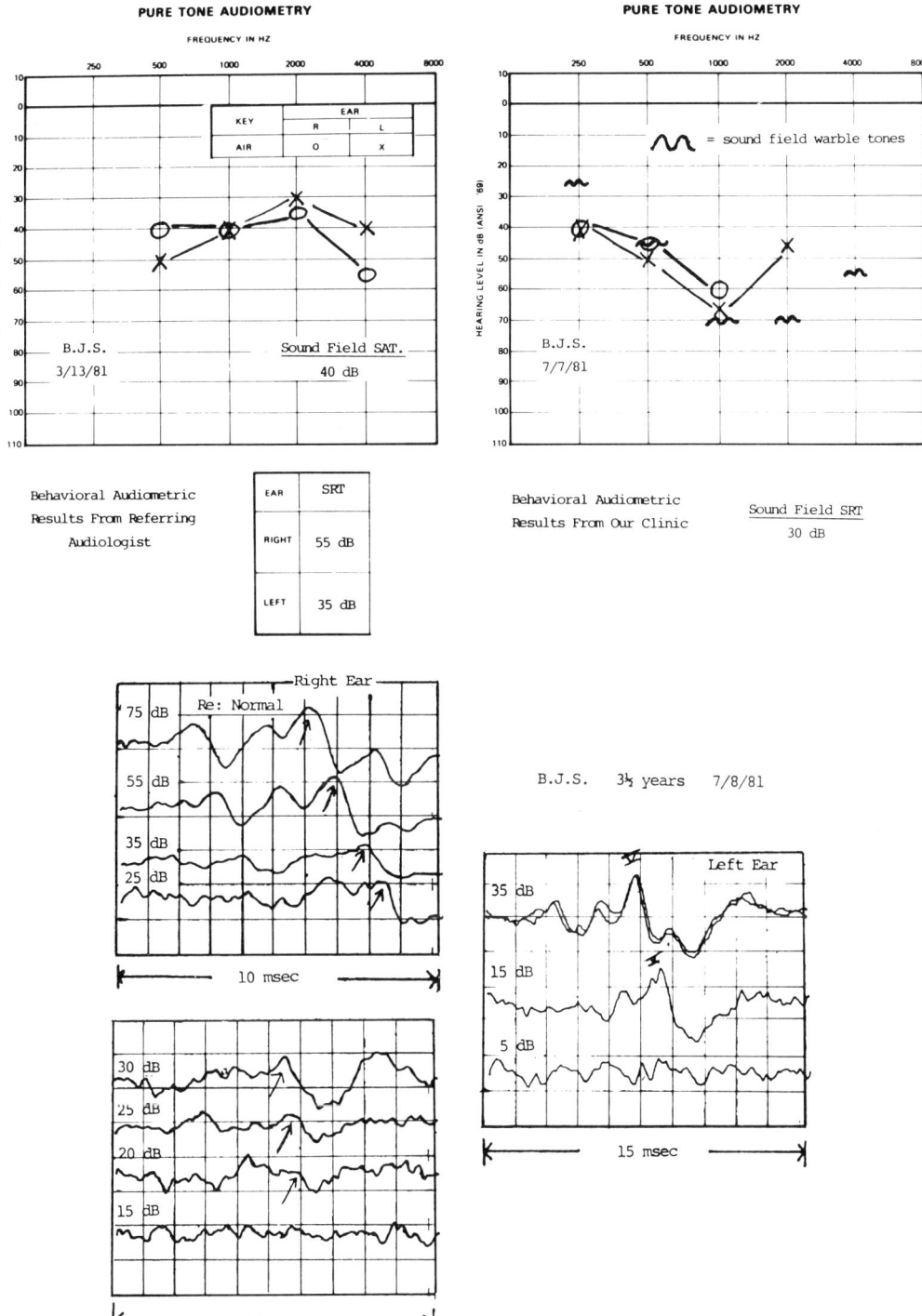

Figure 15.7. A 3-year, 6-month-old girl with generalized developmental delay. She is referred to us prior to fitting a hearing aid with behavioral audiometric results indicating a moderate-to-severe bilateral hearing loss. Our behavioral tests agreed with the referring audiologist. The ABR verifies normal auditory sensitivity for the left ear and mild loss for the right ear confirming the parents observations. Subsequent tympanometry and otological diagnosis revealed right middle ear effusion and a normal left drum.

ometry. In fact, many times ABR provides the only available clinical information on the auditory status of difficult-to-test infants and children. Table 15.3 summarizes the populations of babies and children for whom ABR can provide useful information.

The other major clinical application of ABR is for the identification of retrocochlear disorders. The physiological function of the two sides of the unimpaired human neurological mechanism is incredibly symmetrical. Consequently, ABR is being used to investigate the presence of space-occupying lesions in the auditory nervous system and for the detection of other neurological disorders that often present symptoms similar to vestibular and labyrinthine disease.

Recall that Wave V, or IV–V complex, is the most stable and robust of the VII component waves during the first 10 msec following the introduction of an auditory stimulus to the ear. Thus, Wave V is considered the most clinically useful. The latency of Wave V is determined by stimulus parameters, cochlear function and neural transmission along both the eighth nerve and the brain stem auditory pathways. Consequently, ABR can be especially useful for detecting early eighth nerve lesions by assessing morphology, interaral and interwave latencies, and sometimes, absolute and relative amplitude of the component waves. Table 15.4 summarizes categories of neurological disorders where ABR can provide useful information.

ABR audiometry has other uses. For example, bone-conducted ABR can be used for the differential diagnosis of conductive vs. sensorineural hearing loss in babies and young, difficult-to-test chlideren and in special problems encountered in the adult population (12). We have used ABR in the differential diagnosis of pseudohypoacousis where the patient was feigning a severe-to-profound bilateral hearing loss. It appears to have potential as a screening procedure in the newborn population (2, 13). Undoubtedly, its application will be expanded in the years ahead.

LIMITATIONS

No test is without limitations and ABR is no exception. The need for sedation under medical supervision limits its application to a medical setting for children 6 months to 3 years and older, difficult-to-test children. The degree of hearing loss in patients with a suspected retrocochlear lesion can preclude the application of ABR completely or render the results ambiguous. If an average hearing loss for 1, 2, and 4 kHz exceeds 70 dB HL, there is a good chance that ABR will yield useless information. For this reason alone, ABR will

Table 15.3
Pediatric Populations for ABR

Age	Description
0–3 months	Neonatal intensive care unit High risk register Deaf parents Meningitis
3–24 months	Persistent otitis media Meningitis Sepsis and ototoxic drug therapy Failure to thrive Deaf parents Delayed speech Parental suspicion
24+ months	Developmental delay Learning disability Meningitis Suspicion of CNS disorder Emotional disturbance

Table 15.4
Disorders Associated with Abnormal ABR

Posterior fossa tumors	Stroke/ischemia
Extraaxial	Metabolic/toxic diseases
Intra-axial	Head trauma
Demyelinating processes	Vascular diseases
Developmental diseases	Coma
Degenerative disorders	Brain death

not completely displace the traditional audiological site-of-lesion test battery. Lack of adequate evidence on the effect of stimulus parameters and anatomical origin of component waves somewhat limits the present level of sophistication of ABR interpretation. Finally more convincing evidence on the interpretation of tone pips is needed before we are able to increase our confidence in ABR for determining an audiometric configuration. Thus, ABR should be used in conjunction with more traditional behavioral audiometry with younger children.

SUMMARY

Following 20 years of research and development ABR seems to have taken its place as a respected and valuable procedure in the armamentarium of audiological tests. It is especially useful in assessing the auditory sensitivity of babies, young, and difficult-to-test children as well as for detecting disorders of the CNS. Although much research has been published on the clinical utility of this technique during the past decade, we are certain to witness considerable refinement and diversity in the application of ABR in the years ahead.

References

1. Davis, H. United States-Japan seminar on auditory responses from the brain stem. *Laryngoscope 89*: 1336–1339, 1979.
2. Davis, H. Electric response audiometry: past, present and future. *Ear Hearing 2*: 5–8, 1981.
3. Jewett, D.L., Romano, M.N., and Williston, J.S. Human auditory evoked potentials: possible brainstem detected on the scalp. *Science 167*: 1517–1518, 1970.
4. Sohmer, H., and Feinmesser, M. Cochlear and cortical audiometry conveniently recorded in the same subject. *Israel J Med Sci 6*: 219–223, 1970.
5. Jewett, D.L., and Williston, J.S. Auditory-evoked far fields averaged from the scalp of humans. *Brain 94*: 681–696, 1971.
6. Rowe, J. Normal variability of the brain-stem auditory evoked response in young and old adult subjects. *EEG Clin Neurophysiol 44*: 459–470, 1978.
7. Chiappa, K.H., Gladstone, K.J., and Young, R.R. Brainstem auditory evoked responses. Studies of waveform variations in 50 normal human subjects. *Arch Neurol 36*: 81–87, 1979.
8. Fria, T.J. The auditory brainstem response: background and clinical applications. *Mono. Contemp. Aud. 2*: 1–44, 1980.
9. Amadeo, M., and Shagass, C. Brief latency clinic-evoked potentials during waking and sleep in man. *Psychophysiol 10*: 244–250, 1973.
10. Starr, A., and Achor, J. Auditory brainstem responses in neurological disease. *Arch Neurol 32*: 761–768, 1975.
11. Stockard, J.J., Stockard, J.E., and Sharbrough, F.W. Nonpathologic factors influencing brainstem auditory evoked potentials. *AMJEEG Technol 18*: 177–209, 1978.
12. Mauldin, L., and Jerger, J. Auditory brainstem evoked responses to bone-conducted signals. *Arch Otolaryngol 105*: 656–661, 1979.
13. Schulman-Galambos, C., and Galambos, R. Brainstem evoked response audiometry in newborn hearing screening. *Arch Otolaryngol 105*: 86–90, 1979

CHAPTER 16

Auditory Brain Stem Response (Middle Latency)

Lee A. Harker, M.D.
Patricia Backoff, M.S.

The summed electroencephalographic middle latency responses (MLR, 10–80 msec) to repeated auditory stimuli were described before the temporally earlier auditory brain stem responses (ABR, 0–10 msec), and the MLR are now gaining clinical popularity. This paper reviews some of our experience with the use of the MLR and cites what we believe to be some advantages of this technique over the ABR.

During testing, the evoked EEG activity is amplified and separated into two or three channels for differential filtering and computer processing to allow simultaneous analysis of ABR and MLR data. This has previously been accomplished utilizing specially adapted laboratory equipment including a PDP 12 computer (1). We are now using a Nicolet Pathfinder II unit and commercially available software for similar processing is now available from the Nicolet Corporation.

Our stimulus requires a special note. Each stimulus consists of a click followed in 45 msec by a tone burst; these paired stimuli are given at a rate modulated between 6 and 10/sec (formerly 8 and 12). When we are attempting to determine auditory thresholds, the first stimulus pair is a wide-band click and a 1-KHz tone burst; the second pair is a narrow-band click centered at 2 KHz coupled with a 500-Hz tone burst; and the third stimulus pair is a narrow-band click centered at 4 KHz and a 250-Hz tone burst. When the purpose of testing is to determine the presence or absence of a retrocochlear lesion, only the first stimulus pair is utilized.

The response to these stimulus pairs consists of a series of waves, the most stable and reliable of which are identified as Na, Pa, and Nb. The latencies of those three peaks evoked by the click portion of the stimulus are approximately 13, 26, and 38 msec, and the latencies for the same peaks which are evoked by the temporally delayed tone burst portion of the stimulus approximate 62, 75, and 88 msec. The latencies of the peaks evoked by the tone burst do not change appreciably if the click portion of the stimulus is omitted.

In the past 8 years, our patients undergoing this type of testing have fallen into two groups, reflecting the needs of our clinical setting. The larger group consists mainly of adult patients in whom a retrocochlear mass lesion is suspected; in these patients, the test yields site-of-lesion data. Although ABR is a highly effective means of detecting the presence of such retrocochlear mass lesions, MLR data can supplement the ABR data. It has been our experience that the earliest ABR change seen with vestibular schwannomas is an increased latency in Wave V and at that point, MLR responses are sometimes normal. With increase in the size of the mass lesion, auditory pure tone thresholds worsen, especially in the higher frequencies, and the Wave V response becomes more delayed and finally disappears. The ABR reflects primarily high frequency mediated cochlear information from the basal turn, and the presence of a sensory hearing loss of greater than 65 dB in the 2- to 4-KHz region considerably reduces the reliability or even the presence of such an ABR (2). A dilemma then exists: Is the lack of an ABR reflective of a sensory hearing loss or the presence of a retrocochlear mass lesion?

We have tested 51 patients with confirmed internal auditory canal or cerebellopontine angle tumors. Of these 51 patients, 20 (39%) had no ABR with stimulation of the involved ear by sufficiently loud click stimuli. This percentage of tumor bearing patients who have no ABR falls within the reported range from other studies (3, 4). In 3 of the 20 patients, there was essentially no hearing in the involved ear and no MLR were recorded to ipsilateral stimulation either. In 4 patients, high frequency thresholds were quite good and an ABR should easily have been elicited; in these cases, the MLR was also abnormal. But in the remaining 13 (25%), the absence of the ABR might have been perceived to be due either to the presence of a tumor or to poor hearing thresholds. In all 13 of these tumor-bearing patients, the MLR were grossly abnormal with increased peak latencies and, usually, with decreased amplitude and a rounding of the peaks. Responses to both the wide-band click and 1-KHz tone burst were usually similarly abnormal. Most often, a MLR click response was present even though the ABR click response was lost, suggesting either a greater sensitivity of the MLR click response, or a greater composition of low frequency response elements to the MLR click response. The simultaneous collection of early and middle latency information, while not unduly extending the length of the test, gives us more information to aid in the management of these patients who account for at least one-fourth of our tumor population.

The smaller group of patients in our clinical setting are tested in an attempt to determine auditory thresholds. Over one-half are under 2 years of age, and older individuals are either multiply handicapped or for other reasons, are unable to be adequately evaluated by conventional audiometric testing. By using all three pairs of compound stimuli, we are able to obtain threshold information roughly corresponding to a behavioral audiogram. Because of time limitations, we are not able to use 5- or 10-dB stimulus intensity increments; the stimulus intensity varies by 15–25 dB depending on the individual situation. The first priority of testing is to obtain an estimate of thresholds utilizing binaural stimulation. The second priority is to obtain full audiometric frequency information and the third priority is to obtain data from ear separately. To complete the full test sequence with our equipment requires 80 minutes of data collection. For this reason, sedation is used in children over age 1. Even with young and multiply handicapped individuals, we are able to obtain sufficient information for auditory rehabilitation purposes in over 80% of the patients with a single testing session.

Musiek and Geurkink (5) have recently reported data directly comparing ABR and MLR in response to low intensity click stimuli in normal hearing subjects. While only positive MLR waves were analyzed, they noted the "MLR waves occur with greater frequency at low sensation levels than ABR waves." Our clinical experience with hearing impaired subjects also suggests a greater MLR sensitivity near threshold.

A second, equally important advantage of the MLR is the ability to easily record responses across the entire audiometric frequency range.

CASE 1

A 19-year-old was suspected of having a hearing loss for 2–3 years after a severe bout of epiglottitis. MLR testing showed no responses to stimuli above 1 KHz AS, and above 500 Hz AD. Clear MLR peaks were seen from the left ear at 65 dB HL for 250 Hz stimuli and 90 dB for 500 Hz stimuli, and from the right ear at 80 dB for 250 Hz and 90 dB for 500 Hz stimuli (Fig. 16.1). Time limitations precluded further repetitions at lower intensities. Conventional audiometry was later possible in this child and confirmed the better low frequency thresholds (Fig. 16.2). The detection of the low frequency thresholds has been much easier since the use of the MLR.

CASE 2

An 18-year-old hospitalized mentally retarded lad with a known congenital hearing loss was referred for quantification of the hearing loss. MLR testing showed no response from the left ear and none above 1000 Hz in the right ear. Right ear responses were noted at 98 dB HL for 1000 Hz tone bursts, 90 dB for 500 Hz signals, and 80 dB for 250 Hz tone bursts. Eventually, after sufficient conditioning, conven-

116 Clinical Otology

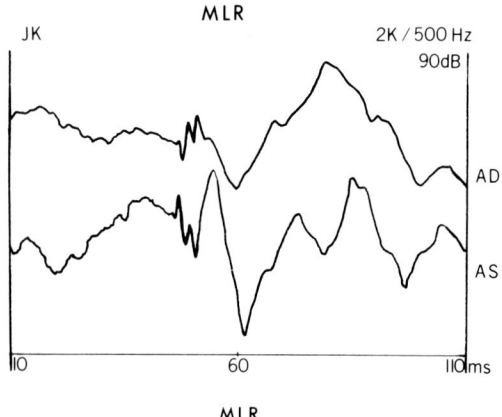

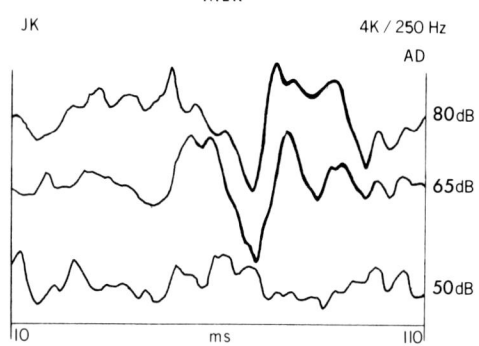

Figure 16.1. MLR from Case 1. No responses are evident in the left half of the traces, where they would normally be identified in response to the 2 KHz (*upper*) and 4 KHz (*lower*) click stimuli. Responses to the low frequency tonal stimuli are seen on the right.

tional audiometry audiometry yielded similar result.

A third advantage of the MLR to the ABR is testing such patients is seen when there is no ABR response. When the peripheral auditory mechanism is nonfunctional in an ear, stimulation of that ear (with appropriate masking of contralateral ear) will evoke neither an ABR nor a middle latency response. No end organ, no neural response. However, when a middle latency response is seen at normal or near normal presentation levels (20–30 dB) and there is no ABR, the auditory periphery must be intact and the function pathology must reside central to that end organ.

CASE 3

A 20-month-old baby was seen for suspected vestibular and auditory abnormalities. The history, physical examination, and functional and radiographic tests led to a diagnosis of intrauterine cytomegalovirus infection. In the right ear (with left ear masking), ABR were seen only at 99 dB HL, whereas they were evident at 30 dB in response to left ear stimulation (Fig. 16.3). But MLR were clearly seen after both right and left ear stimulation at 30 dB with all frequency stimuli (Fig. 16.4). In such a child with multiple handicaps, the presence of normal middle latency auditory responses can be helpful information for the neurologist assessing localized

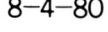

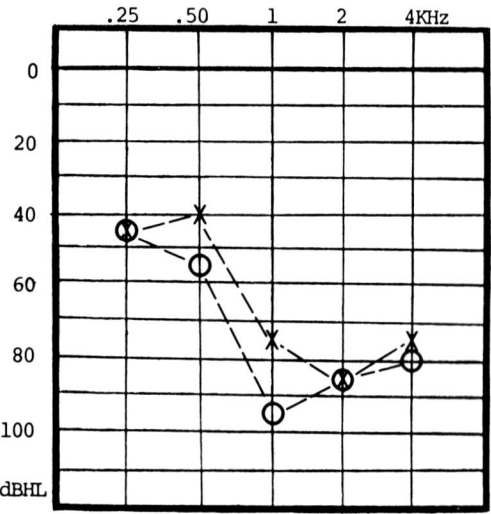

Figure 16.2. Behavioral audiogram from Case 1. See text.

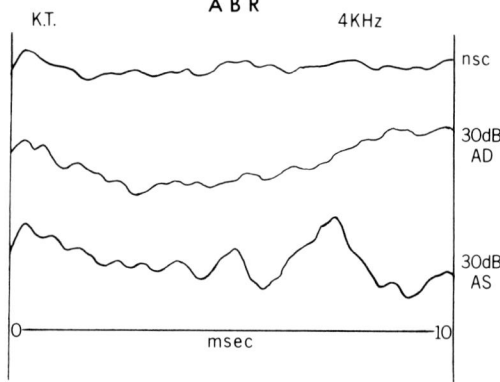

Figure 16.3. ABR from Case 3. Obvious response AS to low level stimulation with none AD.

Middle Latency ABR

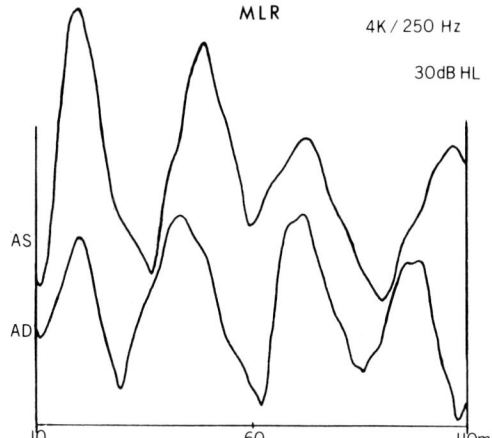

Figure 16.4. Representative MLR from Case 3. Obvious response to click and tone burst stimuli in each ear. Also demonstrates the ease with which low intensity 250-HZ tone bursts can elicit a response.

versus generalized brain damage, and it can be crucial for the rehabilitative audiologist, since high level amplification is not appropriate when low level stimulation of an end organ evokes a normal middle latency response.

The approaching commercial availability of hardware and software to simultaneously gather information from the early and middle components of the auditory responses is gratifying. The ABR has proven to be a powerful tool for site-of-lesion testing; however, its ability to measure hearing threshold sensitivity in young children and adults is frequently overestimated. The increased sensitivity, the ability to easily obtain low as well as high frequency threshold information, the ability to easily obtain low as well as high frequency threshold information, and the assessment of higher level neural function are sufficient benefits for us to continue utilization of middle latency response testing, and to recommend it to others.

References

1. Harker, L. A., and Backoff, P. Middle latency electric auditory responses in patients with acoustic neuroma. *Otolaryngol Head Neck Surg* 89: 131-136, 1981.
2. Brackman, D.E., and Selters, W.A. Brainstem electric audiometry: acoustic neurinoma detection. *Rev Laryngol Otol Rhinol* (Bord) 10J: 49-51, 1979.
3. Selters, W.A., and Brackmann, D.E. Brainstem electric response audiometry in acoustic tumor detection. In *Acoustic Tumors*. Vol. 1. House, W.F. and Luetje, C.M. (Eds). Baltimore: University Park Press, 1979.
4. Clemis, J.D., and McGee, T. Brain stem electric response audiometry in the different diagnosis of acoustic tumors. *Laryngoscope* 89: 31-42, 1979
5. Musiek, F., and Geurkink, N.A. Auditory brainstem and middle latency evoked response sensitivity near threshold. *Ann Otol* 90: 236-240, 1981

CHAPTER 17
Labyrinthine Fistulas

Victor Goodhill, M.D.

Perilymphatic fistulas due to bone or membrane lesions can occur anywhere in the labyrinthine system but especially in the round window niche and/or in the oval window area. In addition to potentially visible "external" fistulas, a variety of intralabyrinthine membrane breaks occur. Among the causes are congenital malformations, necrotizing bone lesions (syphilis and other temporal bone diseases), sequellae of stapedectomy and other otosurgical procedures, physical trauma, and barotrauma.

In some cases, spontaneous healing may occur, as judged by resolution of symptoms. Otherwise, the basic therapy is surgical repair.

CONGENITAL FISTULAS

Congenital round window and oval window malformations with or without fistulas can occur in utero and may persist into infancy, childhood, and adult life.

Microfissures in adult temporal bones include (a) fissure between the posterior canal ampulla and the round window niche, and (b) fissure superior to the oval window between the tympanum and the vestibule. Harada et al. (1) found oval window microfissures in 25% of 331 human temporal bones. Goycoolea et al. (2) have found round window permeability routes in cat experiments. Cochlear aqueduct-perilymph relationships have recently been studied by Bergmann et al. (3).

Congenital round window fistulas due to bone fissures in the round window niche can cause fluctuating mixed hearing loss. The niche may be very wide and the round window membrane may be abnormally exposed, unlike its usual partially "hidden" location. Clear fluid may well up slowly in the niche.

Definitive round window membrane "holes" are exceedingly rare. The most common fistula location is at the inferior periphery of the round window membrane attachment. A large cochlear aqueduct can play an etiological role. This "mix" of cerebrospinal fluid (CSF) and perilymph can also leak into the middle ear via Hyrtl's fissure, a bony cleft inferior to the round window.

Congenital oval window fistulas are due to a variety of anomalies. The stapes itself may be monopod, and/or the oval window periphery may contain congenital bony fissures.

The "fissula ante fenestram" anterior to the oval window is open in the fetus and extends from the middle ear to the labyrinthine vestibule through the otic capsule. It has been observed partly open and partly closed as late as the second year of infancy, and may persist in the adult.

Congenital oval window cysts, perilymph filled "sacs" represent congenital malformations with continuity between the perilymph and cerebrospinal fluid systems. Such fistulas may be discovered at tympanotomy following otitic meningitis with an accompanying unilateral sensorineural hearing loss.

TEMPORAL BONE NECROSIS FISTULAS

The "Hennebert" syndrome refers to eye deviations and/or dizziness resulting from transcanal pneumatic compression and/or rarefaction (4, 5). Originally attributed to syphilis, it can be elicited in nonspecific temporal bone lesions. This is also true of the "Tullio" phenomenon of eye deviation and/or vertigo following acoustic stimulation. There are very few reports of surgically demonstrated luetic fistulas (Fig. 17.1).

Surgical exploration may reveal a fistula resulting from bony dehiscences along the round window membrane attachment. Sealing of such dehiscences with connective tissue (perichondrium or fascia) may result in alleviation of either the vertigo, hearing loss, or both.

Fistulas can occur in both acute and chronic otomastoiditis, with vertigo and spontaneous nystagmus, which may be manifest or detected on ENG examination. ENG with calorization may show a hypoactive or hyperactive response. Mixed conductive and sensorineural hearing loss lesions can occur.

Labyrinthine fistula as a complication of otomastoiditis is most commonly the sequel of keratoma (cholesteatoma), tympanosclerosis, granulomatosis, or polyposis. A common location is in the dome of the horizontal semicircular canal. The fistula may be total, with complete exposure of the perilymphatic space, or subtotal, with bone erosion and only marginal exposure of the perilymphatic space endosteum. In addition, a fistula may occur through the oval window following necrosis of the stapedial arch and footplate, or through the bony cochlear wall. With such a fistula, there may be gradual but occasionally sudden cochlear hearing loss, with tinnitus, and/or vertigo. Such keratoma lesions also occur in the round window niche and may rupture through the round window membrane with fistulization into scala tympani.

Management involves delicate microsurgical bone removal and closure with a tissue graft.

OTOSCLEROSIS SURGERY FISTULAS

Kessel (6), in 1878, in the first surgical oval window opening and stapes extrac-

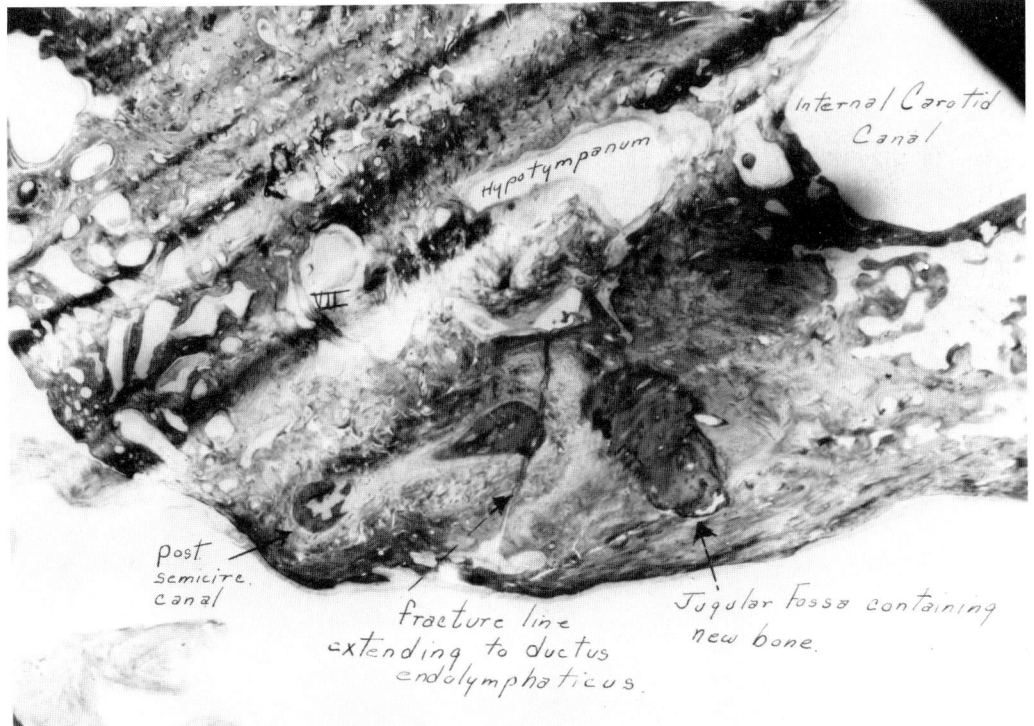

Figure 17.1. Hypotympanum. The two limgs of posterior semicircular canal solidly cast in new bone, from which fracture line diverges, extending to ductur endolymphaticus. Superior level of jugular fossa also contains new bone. VII- seventh nerve. Reproduced from Goodhill, V. (10).

tion in otosclerosis, created a fistula. Miot (7), in 1890, reported a number of successful stapes mobilizations for otosclerosis. Undoubtedly some of his poor results were due to unhealed surgically produced fistulas.

The Lempert semicircular canal fenestration consisted of creation of a fistula which was sealed by a tympanomeatal flap.

In early mobilization techniques by transincudal pressure or by fracturing footplate margins, a temporary or permanent fistula in the oval window was created.

In modern stapes surgery, surgical oval window fistulas are created and covered, hopefully sealed, but the term fistulization has rarely been used in this context.

Both primary and secondary fistulas occur in stapedectomy. A partial or complete conductive loss following stapes surgery, the "backsplash phenomenon", is due to unhealed fistulization (8). Of course, there have been many reports of fistulas causing partial or complete cochlear hearing losses.

Primary perilymphatic fistula following stapedectomy is manifested by a persistent conductive loss in some cases, more commonly by a fluctuating or fixed sensorineural hearing loss.

The most serious sequel is total cochlear hearing loss accompanied by vertigo. Tinnitus is present also in varying degrees.

Complete bed rest for 48–72 hours with head elevated is the first management step. If there is no rapid improvement in hearing and/or vestibular function, surgical exploration and repair is urgently indicated.

Surgical repair involves the following steps: (a) careful and complete removal of prosthesis; (b) removal of fistula mucosal tract, avoiding saccule and utricle; and (c) closure with a tissue graft, preferably perichondrium or fascia (Fig. 17.2).

The sealed oval window may either be left disconnected from the incus temporarily or may be reconnected to the incus, preferably with a cartilage autograft, which will expedite a mucosal seal from oval window to incus.

Preoperative and postoperative antibiotic and steroid therapy is advisable.

TRAUMATIC FISTULAS

Traumatic events which can produce fistulas include: (a) head trauma; (b) blunt ear trauma; (c) penetrating ear trauma; (d) acoustic/blast trauma; (e) tubotympanic compression trauma; and (f) flying and diving barotrauma.

Trauma can cause labyrinthine perilymph fistulas from fractures through oval window, round window, cochlear promontory, and/or semicircular canals. CSF and perilymph fistulas due to internal membrane breaks can coexist (Fig. 17.3).

Surgically visualized perilymph fistulas as seen in the middle ear via promontory fractures or from oval window and/or round window membrane breaks may be accompanied by surgically invisible intralabyrinthine perilymph-endolymph fistulas due to internal membrane breaks. The latter can occur alone. In 1971, I reported three cases of surgically confirmed labyrinthine fistulas in stress related or physical exertion related cases of sudden hearing loss (9). In an additional paper (10), my colleagues and I confirmed the phenomenon of perilymphatic fistulas which can occur in either round or oval or both windows in cases associated with prior physical or barotrauma stresses.

Hydrodynamic (CSF) or *aerodynamic (tubotympanic)* routes (Fig. 17.4) can be responsible for such membrane breaks. They can coexist.

Hydrodynamic Explosive Fistula Mechanisms Via the CSF System

Labyrinthine perilymph-endolymph systems are linked to arterial, venous, and CSF hydrodynamic forces. Crucial CSF-perilymph relationships function either through the cochlear aqueduct or through internal auditory canal neural foramina. Sudden CSF pressure surges to the perilymph system can cause explosive fistulas (Fig. 17.5).

Variations in patency between perilymph-CSF connections, cochlear aqueduct and internal auditory canal are significant (11–16).

Explosive fistulas can result from either self-induced diaphragmatic splinting

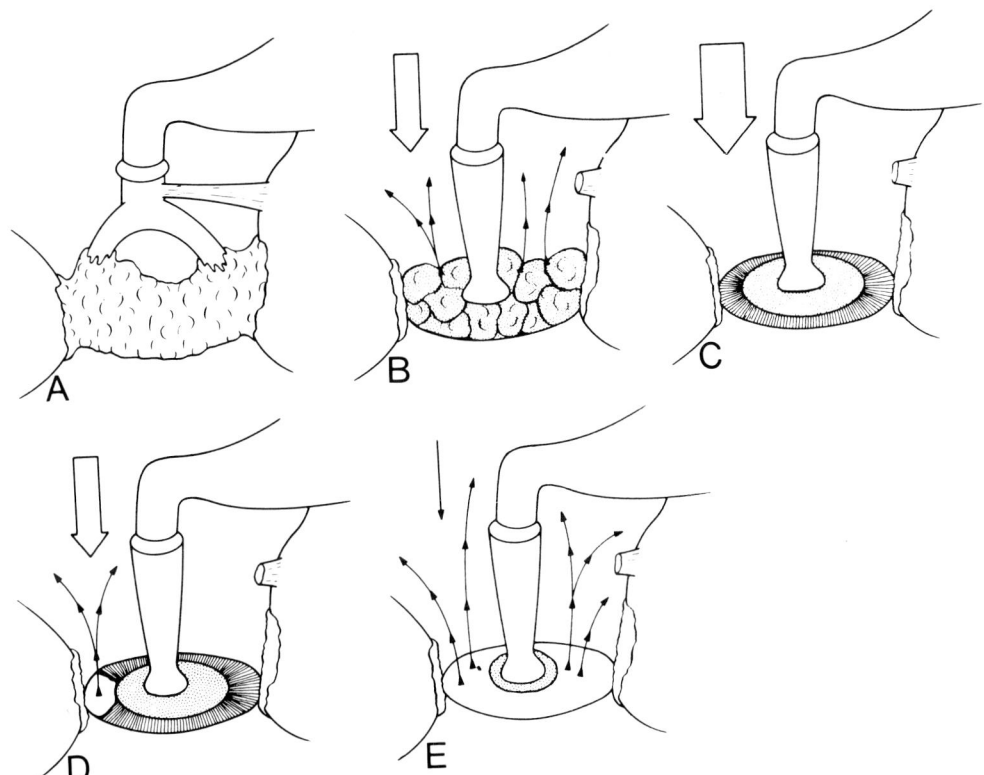

Figure 17.2. Sequence of events from (A) preoperative otosclerotic state (fixed stapes) to (B) first postoperative day, in which a fistula is always present, to (C) final ideal result with completely hermetically sealed oval window-to-incus strut. (D) Partial and major perilymphatic leaks, causing backsplash and partial conductive loss and (E) major backsplash with major conductive loss, indicate relationship between size of fistula and extent of conductive hearing loss. Reproduced from Goodhill, V. (10).

stresses or from other Valsalva forces, environmental barotrauma or head trauma.

The *cochlear aqueduct route to scala tympani* can cause leaks from round window membrane and/or internal leaks through Reissner's, basilar, saccular, utricular, or semicircular canal membranes.

The *internal auditory canal route to scala vestibuli* can cause leaks from oval window via footplate or through anterior oval window ligament, and/or internal labyrinthine membrane breaks producing explosive fistulas.

Aerodynamic Implosive Fistula Mechanisms

Aerodynamic pressure surges via the tubotympanic system communicate with both round window membrane and oval window footplate and ligament areas as routes for *implosive* fistulas (Fig. 17.6). Self-induced forceful Eustachian tube inflation forces or tubotympanic Valsalva forces in flying and diving can cause implosive round window and/or oval window leaks, with chain reaction internal labyrinth membrane breaks (Fig. 17.7).

1. Head Trauma Fistulas. Both closed and open head injuries can produce perilymph leaks. If fractures occur, they may also result in CSF fistulas, via explosive and/or implosive routes. I reported three examples (17).

2. Blunt Ear Trauma Fistulas. Blunt blows to the auricle can produce perilymph fistulas. Open hand slaps to the

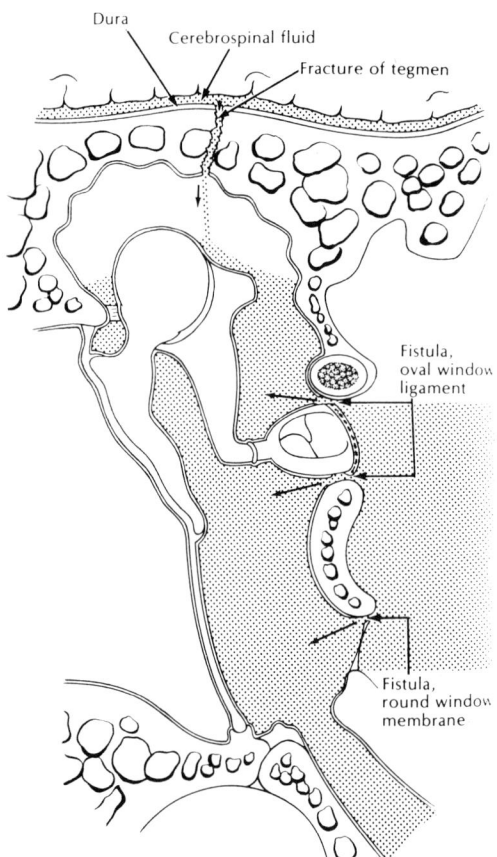

Figure 17.3. Diagrammatic representation of the most common potential pathways for posttraumatic CSF otorrhea: through a tegmental fracture, OW or RW rupture. (From Shulman, in Goodhill).

auricle which usually produce large tympanic membrane perforations may be accompanied by perilymph fistulas. Two illustrative cases were reported by me (17).

3. Penetrating Ear Trauma Fistulas. Gunshot wounds, slag injuries, and iatrogenic injuries in attempts to remove external ear canal and middle ear foreign bodies can be causes of penetrating perilymph leaks which may accompany tympanic membrane-ossicular injuries. Oval window, round window, and intralabyrinthine lesions frequently occur due to labyrinthine capsule fractures.

4. Acoustic/Blast Trauma Fistulas. High intensity acute acoustic trauma (not related to ordinary noise induced hearing loss) and/or blast from explosives can produce perilymph fistulas with or without tympanic membrane ruptures.

5. Tubotympanic Compression Fistulas. Forced "tubal clearing" done voluntarily by violent closed nose blowing can produce perilymph leaks. Miller et al. (18) reported studies on chronic effects of phasic middle ear changes. In high pressure phasic guinea pig experiments, they found round window rupture in 25–50% of animals.

Head (19) reported sudden round window fistula in a diver attempting to clear his ears by a forced Valsalva maneuver.

6. Flying and Diving Barotrauma Fistulas. Oval window and round window fistulas can occur because of pressure changes in flying and diving (20, 21). Schuknecht and Gacek (22) reported a round window marginal linear tear producing severe sensorineural hearing loss in a scuba diver who noted sudden otalgia and deafness at a depth of 12 feet.

SUDDEN HEARING LOSS AND PERILYMPH FISTULAS

Sudden hearing loss can occur as a result of lesions of the external ear, middle ear, inner ear, internal auditory meatus and canal, cerebellopontine angle, and lesions of the central nervous system. Although sudden hearing losses may be conductive or sensorineural, mild or moderate in degree, the emphasis here relates to moderate, severe, or total cochlear losses. Tinnitus and vertigo are frequent concomitants.

Differential diagnosis must include Meniere's disease, labyrinthine complications of previous ear surgery, ear or cranial trauma. In addition, one must consider acoustic trauma, barotrauma, ototoxicity, labyrinthogenic diseases such as syphilis, sudden edema in an eighth nerve tumor, multiple sclerosis, Cogan's syndrome, encephalitis, metastatic carcinoma, and a number of cerebrovascular lesions. Malingering and psychogenic hearing losses must always be considered in the differential diagnosis. Two types of sudden hearing loss occur—idiopathic and perilymphatic fistula (Fig. 17.8).

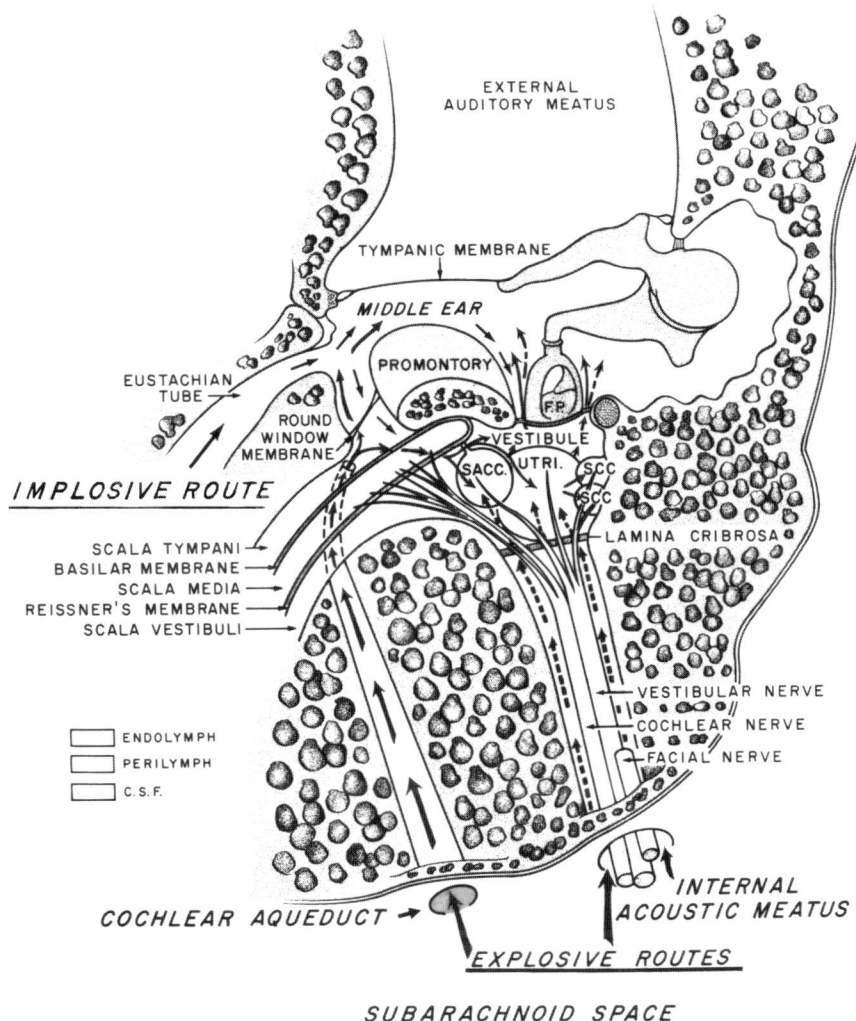

Figure 17.4. Possible pathways of implosive and explosive forces in inner ear. Reproduced from Goodhill, V. (10).

The term idiopathic has been used in discussing the lesion of sudden sensorineural hearing loss occurring in a previously presumably normal ear. Various hypotheses and speculations characterize management based on presumptive viral, vascular, endocrine, allergic, and/or other causes. This therapy has been purely empirical in the past and continues to be so today.

Labyrinth membrane fistulas have been found in cases with barotrauma and physical exertion, in stresses from tubotympanic and/or CSF systems, and without clearcut physical stress histories. Both oval window and round window fistulas occur, as well as associated presumptive intralabyrinthine membrane ruptures (Fig. 17.9).

COMMENTS ON SURGICAL ASPECTS OF FISTULA REPAIR

The appearance of a fistula is not easy to describe. It is not usually a "rapidly running stream." It more commonly appears as a slow limpid clear fluid collection.

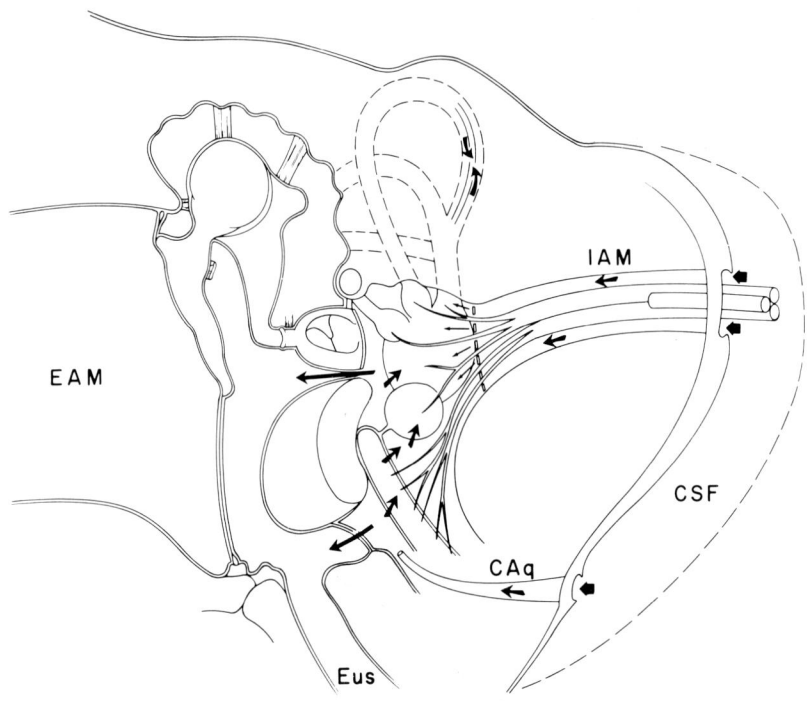

EXPLOSIVE ROUTES

Figure 17.5. Explosive routes for labyrinthine membrane ruptures from CSF system via cochlear aqueduct or internal auditory meatus. Reproduced from Goodhill, V. (10).

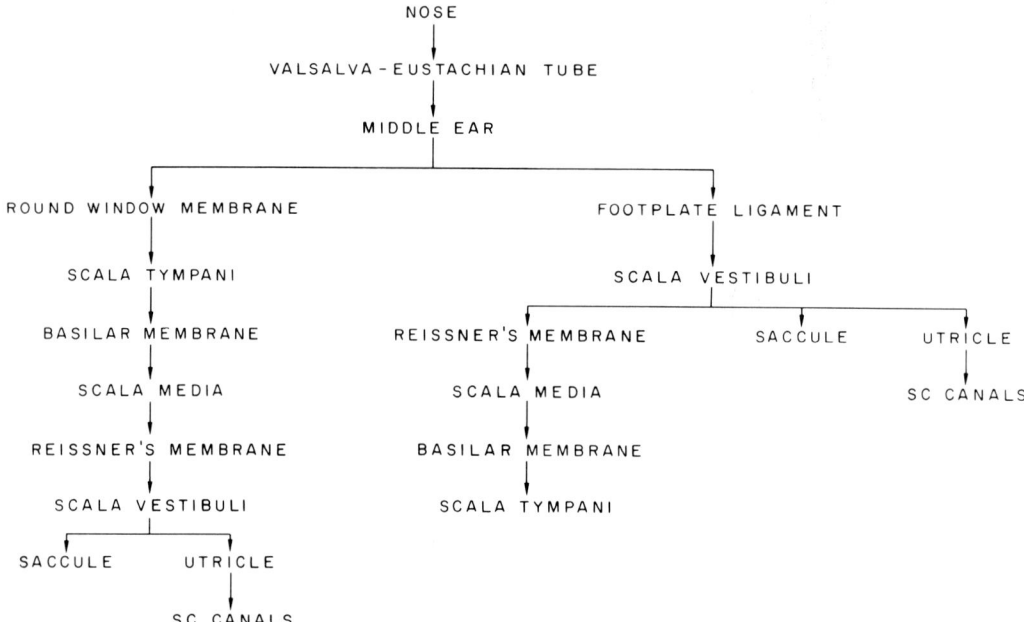

Figure 17.6. Schematic diagram for implosive routes. Reproduced from Goodhill, V. (10).

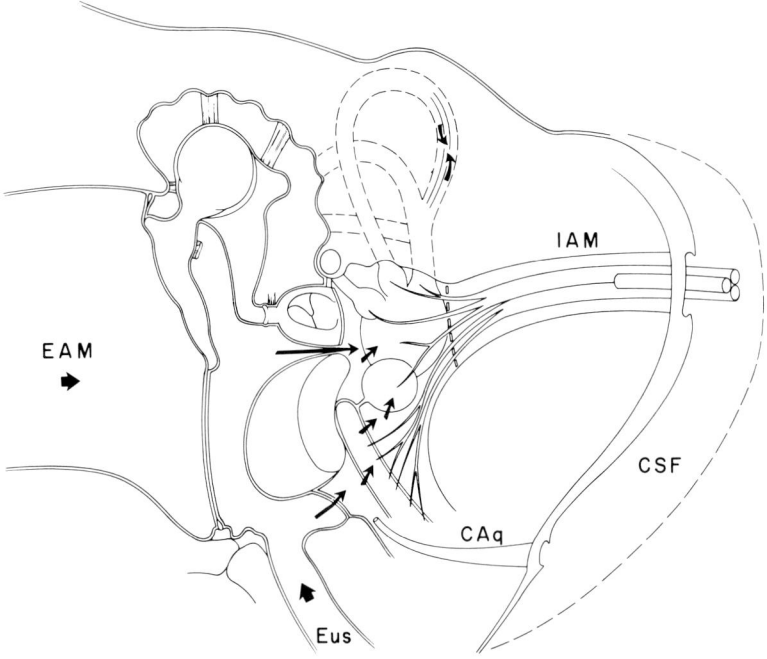

IMPLOSIVE ROUTES

Figure 17.7. Implosive routes for labyrinthine membrane ruptures from middle ear, eustachian tube, and external ear. Reproduced from Goodhill, V. (10).

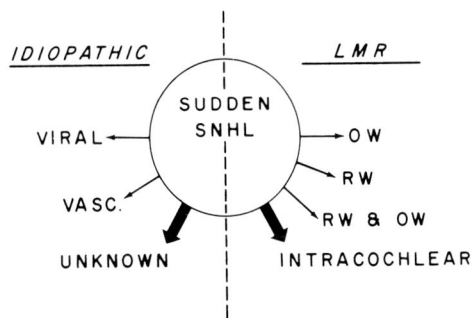

Figure 17.8. Sudden sensorineural hearing loss: idiopathic (viral, vascular, other) and labyrinth membrane rupture (*LMR*) (implosive, explosive) etiologies. *OW*, oval window *RW*, round window. Reproduced from Goodhill, V. (12).

In the oval window niche, it tends to "puddle" anterior to the anterior crus in the region of the fistula ante fenestram. Recurrent seepage follows gentle suction. It rarely occurs posterior to the posterior crus or through a footplate fracture.

In the round window niche, a fistula most commonly occurs at the inferior margin of the round window membrane in the most superior portion of the round window niche. Only a rim of the round window membrane is usually seen. Actual "holes" in the round window membrane are rare. One sees a recurrent seepage of clear fluid at the inferior portion of the round window membrane attachment, with fluid occasionally collecting in the floor of the round window niche.

Fistulas in existence for days or weeks will usually be surrounded by fibrous bands which require microdissection, followed by fine suction.

Leaks may vary from the exceedingly rare "gusher" to a minute persistent flow, which may be increased by gentle incudostapedial joint palpation or jugular compression.

It has not been our practice to drill away

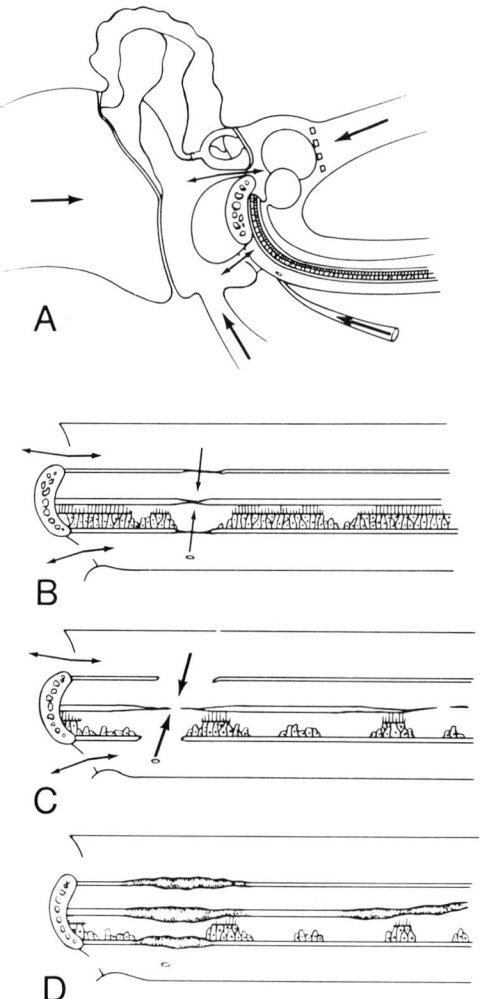

Figure 17.9. Potential labyrinthine sequelae: theoretic possibilities. (A) Diagram of explosive-plus-implosive rupture routes. (B) Minor intralabyrinthine lesion with minimal damage to organ of Corti. (C) Major ruptures with persistent intracochlear fistulae. (D) Healed intracochlear lesions. Reproduced from Goodhill, V. (12).

round window niche bone in attempts to better visualize the round window membrane.

In oval window fistula, endosteum is gently elevated from the margin of the anterior crural region to furnish a base for anchorage of the connective tissue graft, either tragal perichondrium or temporalis fascia. Similarly, in the round window niche region, endosteum is elevated from the superior round window niche bony lip and from inferior round window niche bony margins. Similar tissue grafting is used. Gelfoam is not a seal.

The diagnostic criteria for perilymph fistula exploration have been ably summarized by Singleton et al. (23), in a study using discriminant analysis techniques. They point out the importance of consideration of bed rest for the first 5 days before surgical intervention. In their report, surgical intervention with repair of the fistula by perichondrial grafts provided effective control of vertigo very frequently, more frequently than restoration of hearing. This finding is in agreement with my experience.

SUMMARY

Perilymph fistulas can occur through various temporal bone fracture areas, through labyrinthine membrane ruptures in oval window and round window, through cochlear promontory bone lesions, through semicircular canal erosions, and may be accompanied by intralabyrinthine transmembranous fistulas.

Explosive and implosive routes for traumatic pressure transmissions have been described. Congenital lesions, temporal bone necrosis, otosclerosis surgery, and various types of trauma—all can cause perilymph fistulas.

A high index of fistula suspicion, and a consideration of all of the above possible causes obviously play a role in diagnosis. Management principles and technical principles have been summarized.

References

1. Harada, T., Sando, I., and Myers, E. Microfissure in the oval window area. *Ann Otol Rhinol Laryngol* 90: 174–180, 1981.
2. Goycoolea, M.V., Paparella, M.M., Juhn, S.K., et al. Oval and round window changes in otitis media. Potential pathways between middle and inner ear. *Laryngoscope* 90: 1387–1391, 1980.
3. Bergmann, K., Haupt, H., Scheibe, F., et al. Der Verschluss des Aquaeductus Cochleae fur Perilymphuntersuchungen Am Meerschweinchen. *Arch Oto Rhino Laryngol* 224: 257–265, 1975.

4. Kohut, R., Waldorf, R.A., Haenel, J.L., and Thompson, J.N. Minute perilymph fistulas: vertigo and Hennebert's sign without hearing loss. *Ann Otol Rhinol Laryngol* 88: 153-159, 1979.
5. Nadol, J.B. Positive "fistula sign" with an intact tympanic membrane. *Arch Otolaryngol* 100: 273-278, 1974.
6. Kessel, J. Uber das mobilisieren des steigbugels durch ausschneiden des Trommelfelles, Hammers und Ambosses bei undurchgangigkeit der Tube. *Arch Ohren Nasen Kehlkopfheilkd* 13: 69, 1878.
7. Miot, C. Die la mobilisation de l'etrier. *Rev Laryngol* 10: 49, 1890.
8. Goodhill, V. Conductive loss phenomenon in post stapedectomy perilymphatic fistulae. *Laryngoscope* 77: 1179-1190, 1967.
9. Goodhill, V. Sudden deafness and round window rupture. *Laryngoscope* 81: 1462-1474, 1971.
10. Goodhill, V., Brockman, S.J., Harris, I., and Hantz, O. Sudden deafness and labyrinthine window ruptures. *Ann Otol Rhinol Laryngol* 82: 2-12, 1973.
11. Althaus, S.R. Spontaneous and traumatic perilymphatic fistulas. *Laryngoscope* 87: 364-371, 1977.
12. Goodhill, V. Labyrinthine membrane ruptures in sudden sensorineural hearing loss. *Proc R Soc Med* 69: 565-572, 1976.
13. Palva, T. Cochlear aqueduct in infants. *Acta Otolaryngol* 70: 83-94, 1970.
14. Palva, T., and Dammert, K. Human cochlear aqueduct. *Acta Otolaryngol* (Suppl): 246, 1969.
15. Stroud, M.H., and Calcaterra, T.C. Spontaneous perilymph fistulas. *Laryngoscope* 80: 479-487, 1970.
16. Tonkin, J.P., and Fagan, P. Rupture of the round window membrane. *J Laryngol Otol* 89: 733-756, 1975.
17. Goodhill, V. Traumatic fistulae. *J Laryngol Otol* 94: 123-128, 1980.
18. Miller, J.M., Axelsson, A., and Potter, W. Chronic effects of phasic middle ear pressure changes. *Ann Otol Rhinol Laryngol* 90: 281-286, 1981.
19. Head, P.W. Decompression injuries in the temporal bone. *J Laryngol Otol* 94: 111-116, 1980.
20. Freeman, P., Tonkin, J., and Edmonds, C. Rupture of the round window membrane in inner ear barotrauma. *Arch Otolaryngol* 99: 437-442, 1974.
21. Jaffe, B.F. Vertigo following air travel. *N Engl J Med* 301: 1385-1386, 1979.
22. Schuknecht, H.F., and Gacek, R.R. Surgery on only hearing ears. *Trans Am Acad Ophthal Otolaryngol* pp. 257-266, 1973.
23. Singleton, G.T., Karlan, M.S., Post, K.N., and Bock, O.G. Perilymph fistulas: diagnostic criteria and therapy. *Ann Otol Rhinol Laryngol* 87: 797-803, 1978.

CHAPTER 18

A Sudden Hearing Loss

Maurice Schiff, M.D.

The causes for sudden hearing loss are numerous as can be seen in Figure 18.1.

INFECTION

The most common cause of sudden hearing loss in the viral category of infection are those seen in children. Fortunately, this is almost universally monaural. Most of these cases, some of whom did not have any manifest parotitis, are attributed to the mumps virus. Van Dishoeck (1), studying a hundred cases of sudden hearing loss seen for the first time, found that over 40% of the cases demonstrated viral antibodies. In addition to that, many of us have now seen cases of sudden hearing loss due to serious influenzae viral infections. This is not to be confused with the hemophilus organism. Of the bacterial infections, certainly meningococcal meningitis is one of the most devastating. This very frequently leaves bilateral severe hearing loss. The infections from other bacterial sources which cause involvement of the inner ear may completely destroy one ear but usually do not take both ears simultaneously.

TRAUMATIC

Certainly head injuries have become more common, particularly since the automobile and motorcycle have come of age. There are numerous episodes of sudden loss, particularly if a fracture involves the petrous portion of the temporal bone. Occasionally, there is a fracture through the labyrinth which not only causes hearing loss but considerable vertigo. This can be seen with and without otorrhea or with and without hemotympanum. With such types, there is little one can do to restore the profound hearing loss.

One of the more optimistic aspects of head injuries in a broader sense are those disturbances relative to the rupture of the round or oval window, or both. Dr. Goodhill (2) originally described his findings and a method for handling these problems. What is fortunate is that very often sealing off the ruptured window will give a prompt return of good hearing. What has become more apparent is that there are many causes for round window ruptures which were totally unsuspected previously. Being hit on the head with a ball, the sudden slamming of a door in a well-sealed automobile, scuba diving, or sudden decompression are some episodes of head injury in which proper audiometric studies show that there is not only fluctuation in hearing but very often an inconsistency between speech reception threshold (SRT) and discrimination (PB) scores. In short, a more optimistic and more aggressive approach towards window exploration in surgery should be entertained and should be done early in the course of the disease.

TUMOR FORMATION

Certainly, acoustic neuromas produce hearing loss, but usually it is a progressive, slow, gradual increase. However, there are several reported cases of rather sudden hearing losses and this should be considered when other proper findings are present. The fact that we now have tests such as the brain evoked response which have a high degree of reliability somewhat facilitates the diagnosis in addition to the other battery of tests. Vascular malformations such as glomus tumors, again, usually do not produce this sudden loss. However, all tumor formations should be suspect if there is any evidence of pre-existent malignancy or tumor elsewhere in the body.

CAUSES OF SUDDEN DEAFNESS

1. INFECTION
   A. VIRAL
   B. BACTERIAL
2. TRAUMATIC
   A. HEAD INJURY
   B. RUPTURE OF OVAL OR ROUND WINDOW
3. TUMOR FORMATION
   A. ACOUSTIC NEUROMA
   B. VASCULAR MALFORMATIONS
4. POSTOPERATIVE
   A. EAR SURGERY
   B. COMPLICATIONS FROM OTHER FAR DISTANT SURGERY
5. PREGNANCY
6. ENDOLYMPHATIC HYDROPS
7. METABOLIC
   A. OTOTOXIC DRUGS
   B. DISTURBANCES OF LIPID METABOLISM
8. VASCULAR
   A. ASSOCIATED WITH HYPERTENSION AND/OR DIABETES
   B. ARTERIOSCLEROSIS
   C. ALTERATIONS IN BLOOD COAGULATION
   D. VASCULITIS, INDUCED OR IMMUNOLOGIC

Figure 18.1

POSTOPERATIVELY

Postoperatively, almost every ear surgeon has had episodes of sudden hearing loss. There is a regular statistical occurrence independent essentially of the technique and the surgeon that occurs for some unknown reason in a very small percentage of cases. Those which occur with cholestatoma and destructive otological disease are better understood. Those which occur occasionally after a stapedectomy are less well understood and the disappointment is considerable both to the patient and the physician.

MENIERE'S DISEASE

Endolymphatic hydrops, or Meniere's disease, is the dilemma of the otologist. The number of forms that this disease can take are many. The usual progress is a very slow, recurrent episode with greater progressive hearing loss, yet there are documented cases of a very rapid, progressive hearing loss only with one or two episodes and a profound loss following these. This problem is also one of the stimuli for the greatest amount of investigation that goes on in otological research. Next to the pursuits of the general category of sensorineural hearing loss, or degenerations, Meniere's probably sits in the back of each investigator's mind as he works out his various research models. Over the years, we have now been able to separate some of the provocative factors in Meniere's disease such as those due to metabolic disturbances, hormonal disturbances, or allergic conditions. Still, the vast majority remain a dilemma.

METABOLIC

The metabolic disturbances of the inner ear are pronounced when considering the toxicity of the amino glycosides. The ototoxic capabilities of many drugs, such as streptomycin, tobramycin, and others are well known. The ototoxic characteristics of such diuretic substances as ethacrynic acid (Edecrin) and furosemide (Lasix) are well known to the otologist but apparently less well known to the internist who uses these highly efficacious drugs. Our colleagues are most happy to comply, when possible, with the removal of these drugs from therapy. Most have not been aware of the ototoxic proclivity they possess.

When one thinks of metabolic diseases, one can certainly include these with various types of hyperlipidemia. One of the audiograms correlated with the chemistries show how high a lipid count can be. The therapy was to quickly lower blood triglycerides from 638 mg%. It brought about dramatic changes in the PB and SRT scores. In one case, the SRT was 75 dB on a given date, and the PB score was 68%. Twelve days later, having been treated with lipid-mobilizing substances as noted in the vascular discussion, the scores reverted to a 0 SRT and 96% PB score. Spencer (3) brought our attention to this in his discussion of hyperlipoproteinemias in the etiology of inner ear disease. I think that his observations were valid and worthwhile. Efforts should be made to correct lipid disturbances in order to maintain not only the inner ear but the general improved vascular state.

Probably one of the substances which should be discussed, since it affects the metabolism greatly, is tobacco. The role of tobacco can find its analogy very readily in the opthalmic literature regarding tobacco amblyopia, or blindness. The otologist is aware of the vasoconstrictor effect produced by tobacco and, likewise, those that occur with coffee and tea, but the role tobacco plays is so aggressive and strong that it is a difficult substance to neutralize other than removing it from the system by abstaining.

VASCULAR

The hearing losses which occur with hypertension and diabetes may very well manifest a sudden episode of hearing loss which may or may not be recoverable depending upon how well controlled the primary disease state is. Those due to arteriosclerosis are more difficult since they represent changes in the central nervous system vessels which are difficult to approach. However, one should not be that pessimistic until an attempt has been made to determine whether or not there is some disturbance of the carotid circulation which very often is amenable to corrective vascular surgery. This is something that should be kept in mind not only for the obese and hyperlipidemic patients but also for those who have the other otological symptoms of vertigo and tinnitus. It has been shown by Jaffe and Penner (4) that viral infections lead to hypercoagulability of blood. This should be kept in mind as a neutralizing effort is made when hearing loss is presented. Prolongation of the prothrombin time by the judicious use of aspirin is something within the knowledge and armamentarium of the otologist and, also, serves a good purpose in many febrile viral states.

In 1974, Schiff and Brown (5) published a series of cases treated with ACTH gel (Acthar) and heparin to show what happened in sudden hearing loss (Fig. 18.2 A-D). First of all, other types of hearing loss had already been considered and either ruled out or tested for and thought to be improbable. This leaves a large pool of ideopathic cases, very often those seen and treated by two or three colleagues previously. It is extremely difficult to have a controlled experimental model. With the discussion as to the mechanism for the action of these drugs is a plea for redefinition of a time frame which will separate those types of sudden hearing loss which can be considered to have been helped by the physician and his treatment or those which Nature has brought about. This author has arbitrarily taken a 30-day period. Within this time frame, there must be moderate or significant hearing improvement; otherwise, the therapy is considered to be of no significant value.

The concept behind the use of these two selective drugs is in the immunological sphere. Much work is going on throughout the world in searching for immunological causes relating to inner ear disturbances. The Japanese were able to demonstrate immune responses in the inner ear. This was presented before the Barany Society in 1975.

Prior to that time, our series of cases were treated based on the hypothesis that an immunological disturbance was occurring either due to some unknown substance provoking change in the inner ear, or possibly a specific anticochlear antigenic substance possibly due to some previous injury. With this concept in mind, the patient was treated with heparin in doses of 10,000 units subcutaneously 2 or 3 times a week, and ACTH 40 units per cc intramuscularly 2 or 3 times a week. The patient was appraised concerning side reactions, which for heparin are very few, except those of sustaining injury soon after the injection. The half-life of heparin is about 4 hours and the premise of its action is not based upon anticoagulation. If this were the case, a much larger dose would have been given and been given more frequently. The side reactions to ACTH are several and, although usually not incapacitating, such as sour stomach or stomach problems, bring a prompt cessation of treatment with ACTH. There is very often a small amount of cool perspiration not of any great consequence. Sometimes there is an alteration in the sleep pattern, both improved sleep or a decrease in the capacity to sleep depending upon the brain chemistry of the individual. Some people feel elevated and others feel depressed. For this reason, after each injection and especially emphatically after the first injection, the patient is required to write notes on these symptoms. If any of these notes indicate adverse reactions, we would arrest the continuation of the treatment. On a few occasions, the ACTH was discontinued. This treatment usually runs only for a period of about approximately 3 weeks. The audiogram is then repeated. If no improvement occurs within 3 weeks, the treatment is discontinued. An audiogram is repeated at the end of the entire treatment period. One of the interesting observations made by patients as they write their notes, and repeated emphatically, is that the head noise tends to get less as the hearing improves. This is probably the most singular subjective symptom that the patient notices first. Likewise, vertigo, which is present occasionally, often comes to an end. A discussion relating to the role of these drugs in vertigo was presented at the Barany Society meeting. Figures 18.2 and 18.3 show the proposed mechanism for the action of the ACTH. This involves the cyclic AMP system. ACTH results in an increase in cyclic AMP. Cyclic AMP has been noted to have several effects which may very well act in this perplexing problem. There is a considerable increase in lipolysis as well as a decrease in platelet aggregation. This is due to the fact that keeping the AMP in the cyclic form decreases the general ADP, which is one of the sticky substances that makes platelets agglutenate.

ACTH

In 1974, references (5) were made to the various actions of ACTH and heparin which will be briefly summarized herein.

A. ACTH is a known stimulant to corticosteroids from the adrenals. This is one of its major functions.

B. It suppresses the antibody antigen reaction, but it does not inhibit its response. The union of antigen and antibody is not prevented, nor is the release of histamine from the sensitized cells prevented. Its major benefit is attributed to suppression of the inflammatory response after cellular injury.

C. ACTH has a distinct lipolytic effect activated by a specific lipase enzyme system. Blood is cleared of chylomicra rather promptly.

D. By altering the amount of available AMP to be regenerated into ADP because of the increase in cyclic AMP, there is a less sticky ADP available.

HEPARIN

A. In brief, heparin exerts its anticoagulant effects specifically as an antiprothrombin action which inhibits the conversion of prothrombin into thrombin. It does not thin blood, nor does it alter the sedimentation rate as often implied.

B. Heparin is a marked stimulus for specific lipoprotein lipase formation. This is so prompt that the blood clearing of lipids from the smaller capillary walls is possible in so short a period of time as 10 minutes. The lipolytic effect is observed at a considerably lower concentration than that used to prolong clotting time.

C. Probably most important is that heparin inhibits the effect of the antibody antigen reaction as noted by Dragstedt (6) over 30 years ago. The fact that heparin complexes and binds histamine quantitatively means that the histamine is now unavailable for cytotoxix purposes. This was demonstrated by Eyring and Dougherty (7) in 1955 and re-emphasized by Dougherty and Dolowitz (8) in 1964. The heparin prevents the histamine from carrying the sodium across the cell membrane into the interior of the cell, therefore damaging the internal mechanism of the cell. This binding of histamine by heparin limits the cyto-destructive effect to the benefit of the capillary with its endothelial and other responsive cells.

D. Heparin is one of the highly sulfated mucopolysaccharides of the ground substance and acts as a cation exchanger and complexes many basic amines and poly-

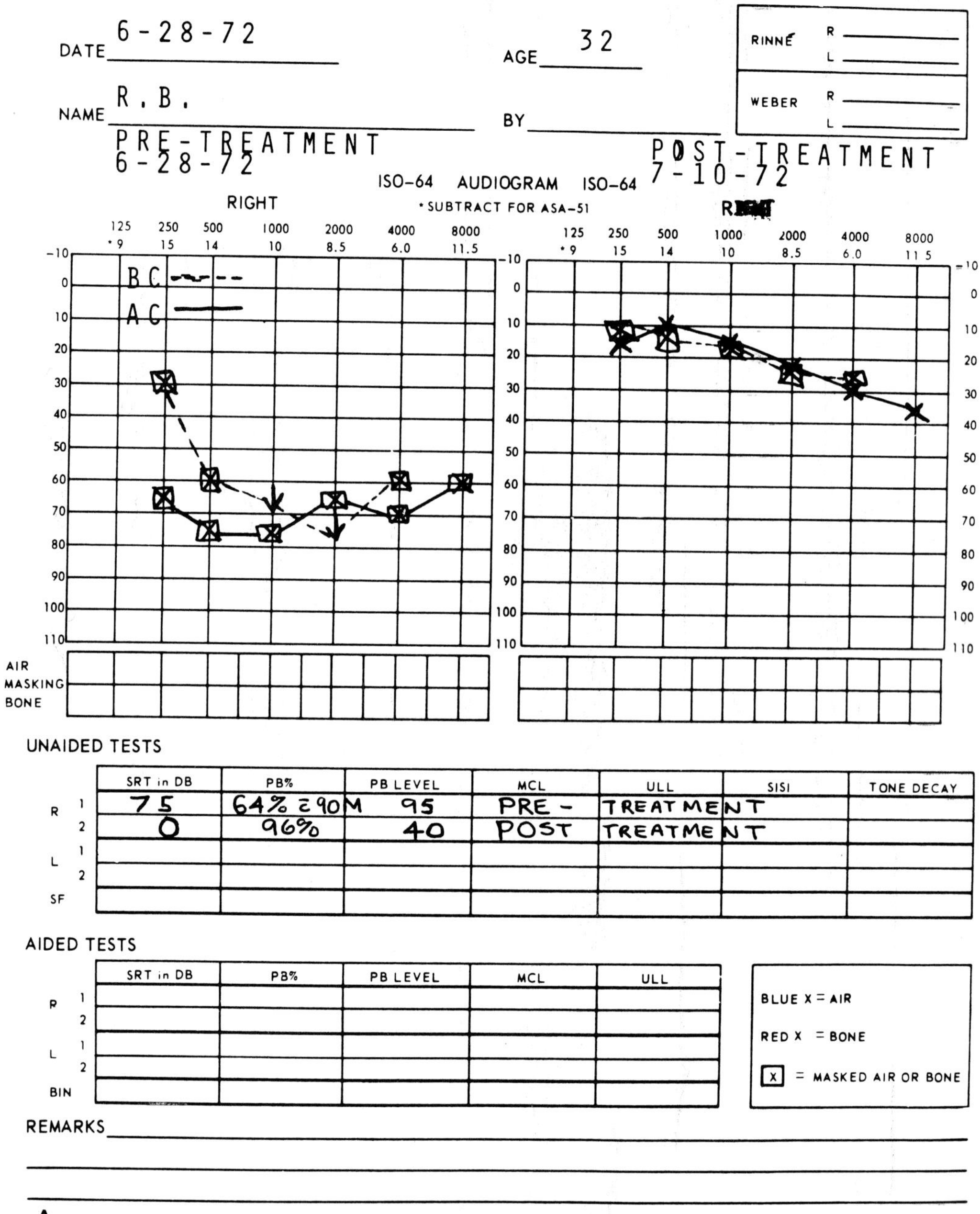

132 Clinical Otology

Figure 18.2 A–D

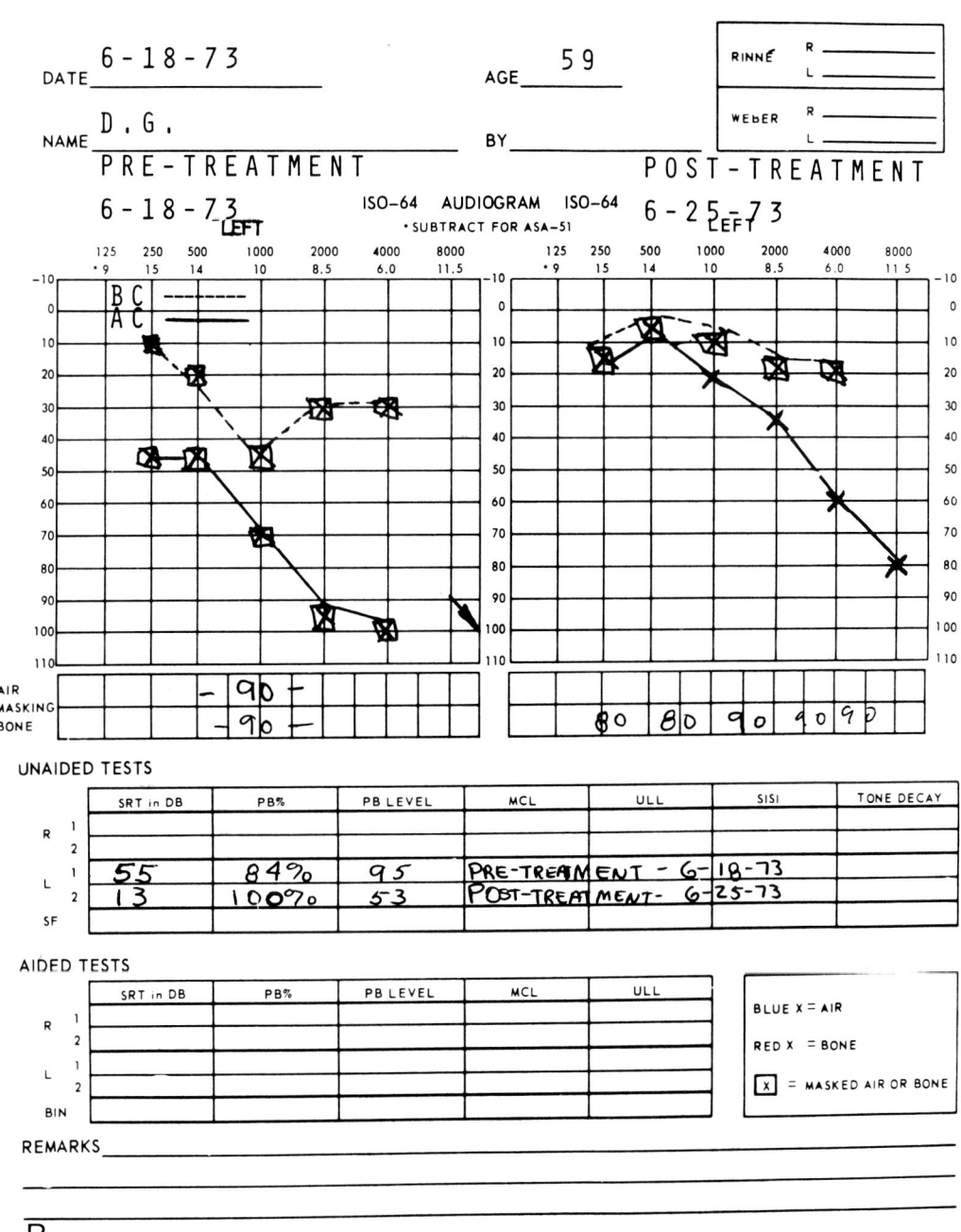

Figure 18.2B

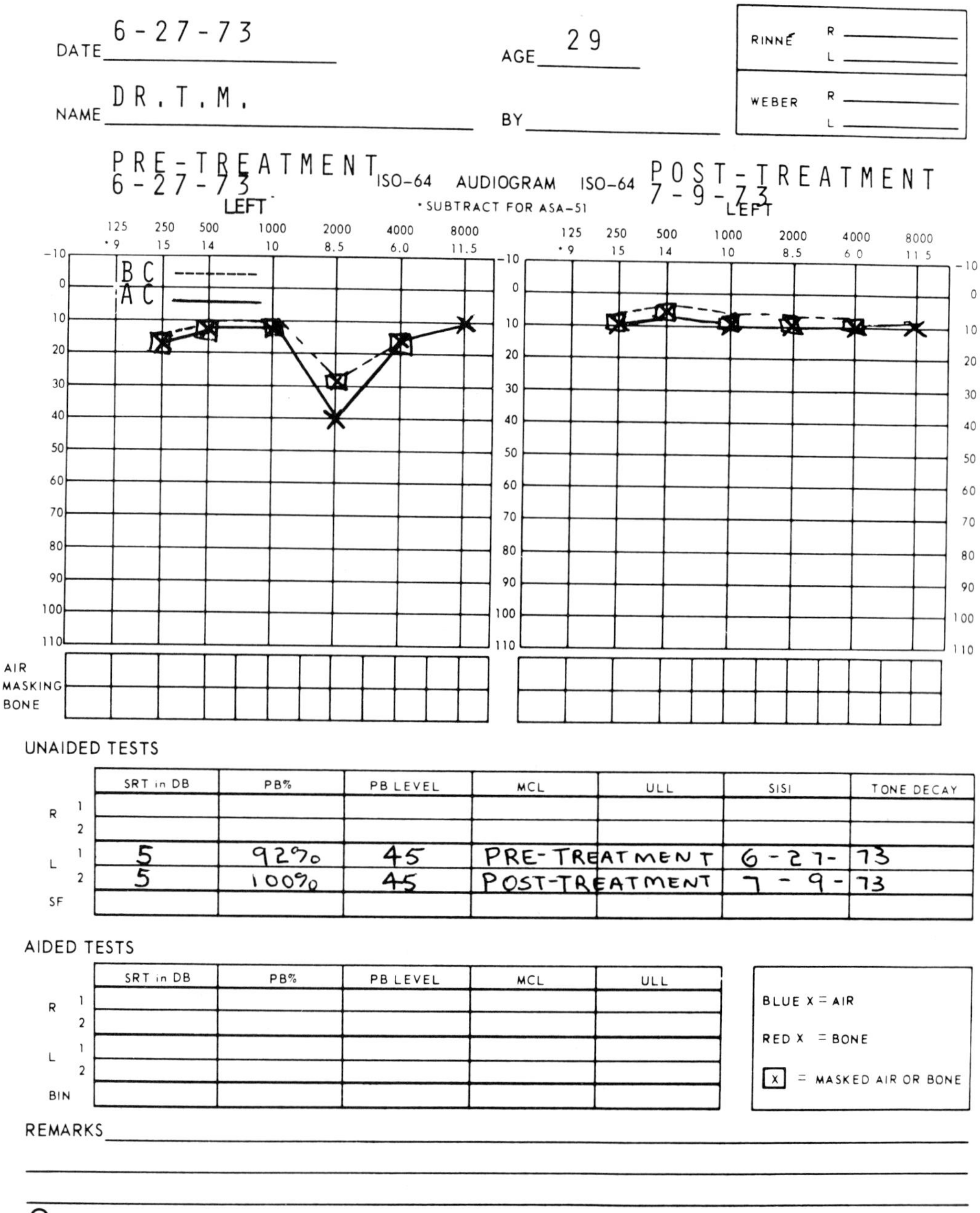

134 Clinical Otology

DATE 6-27-73 AGE 29

NAME DR.T.M. BY

RINNE R ___ L ___
WEBER R ___ L ___

PRE-TREATMENT 6-27-73 LEFT ISO-64 AUDIOGRAM ISO-64 POST-TREATMENT 7-9-73 LEFT
*SUBTRACT FOR ASA-51

BC ----
AC ——

UNAIDED TESTS

		SRT in DB	PB%	PB LEVEL	MCL	ULL	SISI	TONE DECAY
R	1							
	2							
L	1	5	92%	45	PRE-TREATMENT		6-27-73	
	2	5	100%	45	POST-TREATMENT		7-9-73	
SF								

AIDED TESTS

		SRT in DB	PB%	PB LEVEL	MCL	ULL
R	1					
	2					
L	1					
	2					
BIN						

BLUE X = AIR
RED X = BONE
☒ = MASKED AIR OR BONE

REMARKS ___

C

Figure 18.2 C

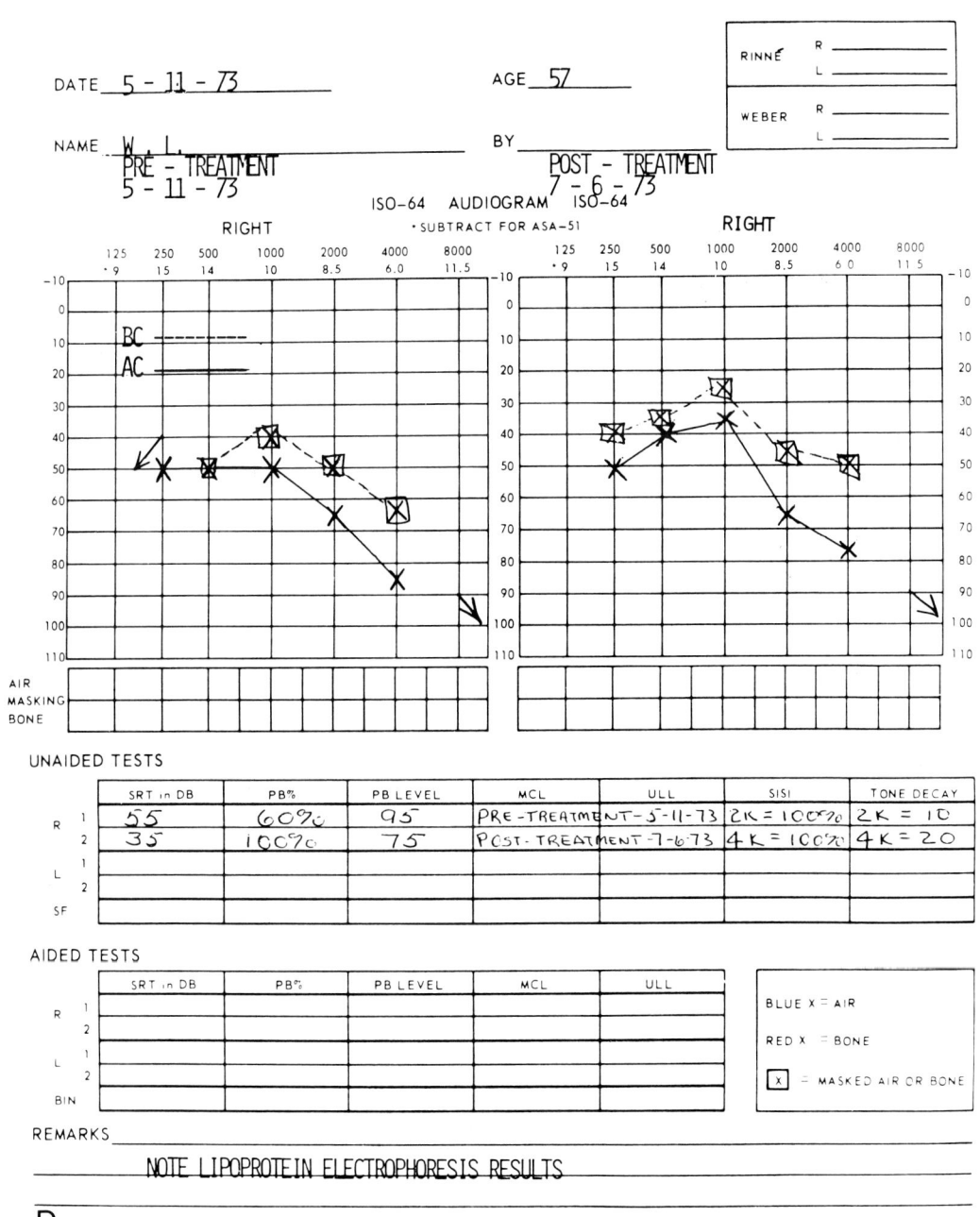

Figure 18.2*D*

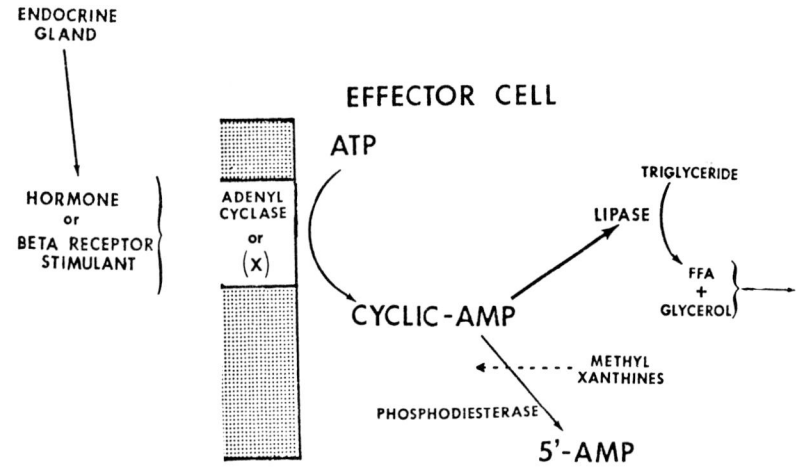

Figure 18.3

peptides. By this mechanism it not only has an anti-inflammatory effect but also an antitoxic effect.

In short, heparin prevents the damaging effect of histamine before it gets started and also limits the amount of degranulation of the mast cells while ACTH decreases the results of the reaction after it has already taken place. Considering this two-pronged approach for specific types of sudden hearing loss, this treatment should be seriously considered. A short time frame is the criterion for any success.

References

1. Van Dishoeck, H.A.E. Sudden perceptive deafness and viral infection. Ann Otol 66: 963–980, 1963.
2. Goodhill, V. Sudden deafness and round window rupture. Laryngoscope 81: 1462–1474, 1971.
3. Spencer, J.T. Hyperlipoproteinemia in the etiology of inner ear disease. Laryngoscope 83: 639–678, 1973.
4. Jaffe, B.F., and Penner, T.A. Sudden deafness associated with hypercoagulation. Trans Am Acad Opthal Otolaryngol 72: 774–778, 1968.
5. Schiff, M., and Brown, M. Hormones and sudden deafness. Laryngoscope 84: 1959–1981, 1974.
6. Dragstedt, C.A. Inhibitory effect of heparin upon histamine release by trypsin, antigen and proteose. Proc Soc Exptl Biol Med 51: 191, 1942.
7. Eyring, H., and Dougherty, T.F. Molecular mechanisms in inflammation and stress. Am Scient 43: 457, 1955.
8. Dougherty, T.F., and Dolowitz, D.A. Physiologic actions of heparin not related to blood clotting. Am J Cardiol 14: 18–24, 1964.

CHAPTER 19
Autoimmune Inner Ear Disease

Brian F. McCabe, M.D.

The author proposes the existence of a new entity, autoimmune sensorineural hearing loss, on the basis of diagnostic study and treatment experience with a series of 18 patients. In each case, the clinical pattern did not fit with known entities and, thus, seemed to merit distinctive categorization. In the one patient in whom tissue was available, a vasculitis was evident, a feature of autoimmune disease. All patients responded to treatment for an autoimmune disease, namely, chronic cortisone and cyclophosphamide therapy.

This condition can be fairly well distinguished from other sensorineural deafnesses in terms of its age of incidence and time-course. This condition in this series of 41 patients involves only those in their 20's and 30's, and is fairly rapidly progressive, unlike sudden deafness (over a few hours) or cochlear otosclerosis or congenital recessive deafness (over years). It is important for otolaryngologists to be able to recognize this disease because *it is one of the few forms of sensorineural deafness for which we have a treatment.*

Two-thirds of patients have had a severe bilateral canal paresis but balance complaints are minor because of their youth and relatively slowly progressive symmetrical loss. Six patients have had a peripheral facial paralysis early in their disease which was temporary. Three patients had middle ear effusions and myringotomies and in all three patients, a dead ear resulted. *Myringotomy in this disorder is absolutely contraindicated.* The effusion will rapidly clear on medical treatment without loss of inner ear function. Laboratory tests are normal except for positive ANA test in most (not all) patients, a high sedimentation rate, and a positive lymphocyte inhibition assay. In the latter test, the suspect's lymphocytes are challenged by prepared inner ear antigen from material harvested in translabyrinthine operations such as acoustic neuroma resection. Eight patients in this series have subsequently manifested other autoimmune diseases, including Cogan's syndrome, chronic ulcerative colitis, rheumatoid arthritis, and Hashimoto's struma.

Physical examination of the tympanic membranes of one patient early in the disease was of particular interest. Both were thickened and immobile, but the right tympanic membrane was most unusual. A large blood vessel coursed from the annular ligament area posteroinferiorly, up and forward across the umbo, into the opposite quadrant. This vessel was observed periodically. The most astounding feature of all was that after completion of treatment (cyclophosphamide and dexamethasone) over 6 weeks, the vessel had disappeared. There is no blood vessel coursing along this route normally. This is a clear example of neovascularization, wherein an organ already supplied by vessels is supplied in a new way in the absence of prior destruction. This is characteristic of granulomatous diseases, a number of which are autoimmune in nature, the clearest example being lethal midline granuloma.

Tissue for pathological examination is very hard to come by in such patients and would be extremely valuable in search for vasculitis. We have only one such tissue sample, in a patient whose disease involved the middle ear and mastoid. The tissue from this patient clearly demonstrated not only vasculitis but also the ghosts of blood vessels which are in the end stages of vasculitis, rings of scar tissue in the granulomatous substrate. This was one of our first patients and was many months into her illness before we thought to start immunosuppressive therapy, after which she healed and has remained so.

Treatment has consisted of a combination of cyclophosphamide and high dose steroids. The former is given intravenously at a level of 2 mg/kg daily over 2 weeks, followed by a rest period of 2 weeks, then a final 2 weeks of infusions. The steroid used has been dexamethasone, 16 mg/day divided, over a minimum period of 6 months. Then a long taper is introduced. If the hearing drops, the steroid is restored to prior levels for an additional 6 months, etc. The longest treatment period has been burned out. The results of treatment have been gratifying. In patients with relatively minor losses, in the range of 30–50 dB, normal or low normal hearing has resulted. In most patients, however, the loss was major, in the 80–100 dB range and in these, the result was stabilization at a 20–30 dB improvement and rehabilitation with a hearing aid. No patient failed to improve and stabilize, and go off medications.

CHAPTER 20

Single Electrode Cochlear Implantation: A Co-Investigator Report

Charles M. Luetje, M.D.
Donald L. Lawrence, Ph.D.

Since August 31, 1979, the author has implanted 9 patients with the single electrode cochlear implant as designed by William F. House, M.D. of Los Angeles. The patients ranged in age from 22-61 years at time of implant. Five were females and 4 were males. The patients had been profoundly deaf from 18 months to 25 years before implant.

The cause of hearing loss was otosclerosis in 4 patients, meningitis in 2, and acquired, unknown in three. Seven patients are users, 2 are in process. In process means implanted, undergoing a 2-month healing period, awaiting the external coil and stimulator unit. There are no nonusers. No complications have occurred.

Data provided by the House Ear Institute regarding average performance of typical cochlear implant wearers on monosyllabic, trochee, spondee (MTS) words and environmental sounds test is presented. Comparison can be made with these scores from the House Ear Institute and those obtained from patients undergoing rehabilitation with their cochlear implant from the Midwest Ear Research Institute.

The authors are part of one of the co-investigator teams associated with the House Ear Institute (HEI). Fourteen such teams in the United States and four in foreign countries have implanted one or more patients each as of April, 1981.

Overall assessment of 7 patients indicates general improvement in the quality of life, abundant accounts of rediscovering and relearning environmental sounds, and objective audiometric data substantiating hearing improvement.

In April, 1979, approximately 20 otologists from the United States were invited to Los Angeles for an intensive 2-day symposium and to become co-investigators in the cochlear implant program as designed by William F. House, M.D., as principal investigator (1). The invitation and symposium were under the auspices of what is now HEI. Clinical trials by Dr. House and members of his staff had established the efficacy of cochlear implantation for postlingually deafened adults. In order to establish a broader base of investigation and complication of data, the otologists were selected from various geographic locations around the United States. Two other surgeons had already implanted patients and had become co-investigators.

By computerizing data from various surgeons located around the United States, the investigative study could be intensified and standardized information used to broaden the base of clinical material.

This paper presents information and data from one of the co-investigator teams. It reviews the formation of this co-investigator team, the audiological evaluation and surgical selection of patients, the rehabilitation of patients after cochlear implantation, and the case material upon which this paper is based.

ESTABLISHING AN IMPLANT PROGRAM

The essential members of our cochlear implant team include an audiologist, a psychologist, a surgical nurse, and an otologist. In addition to an audiological educational background, our audiologist has taught audiology, organized and presided over various parent deaf education groups, and is rather proficient in mechanical and electronics repair. This diversity overlaps into some of the areas of rehabilitation and maintenance of various components of the cochlear implant system.

The psychologist on our team is in private practice with another group of psychologists located several miles from our office. This has not posed a problem nor do we anticipate one. Prospective cochlear implant patients who have been selected for surgery based upon audiometric, vestibular, and radiographic data undergo psychological evaluation to assess cognitive abilities, personality and mental status, and motivation. The psychologist establishes whether the patient meets the following criteria for cochlear implantation:

1. no evidence of severe organic brain damage;
2. no evidence of psychosis;
3. no evidence of mental retardation;
4. no personality traits that would make program completion unlikely;
5. no unremitting, unrealistic expectations of the cochlear implant.

The surgical nurse is the stabilizing coordinator of the entire program. She coordinates all of the audiometric, vestibular, radiographic, and psychological testing and arranges dates for each of these. She receives the information packets that come from the HEI and corresponds with the patients making certain they understand how to fill out various questionnaires and other information pertinent to receiving the cochlear implant. She verifies that the hospital has received the cochlear implant packages containing the internal and external coils, stimulator unit, and all of the other items. She coordinates the surgical date with the operating room and is the one to whom we all turn for seeing to it that the entire procedure runs smoothly.

The otologic surgeon sees the patient initially with basic audiometric data. The initial interview is probably the most important. The surgeon must decide if the patient is a surgical candidate based upon the etiology and the amount of hearing loss. It is at this interview and examination that the patient and family express their concern regarding the specific difficulties the hearing loss creates for them. The surgeon must allow time and create an atmosphere of concern and understanding to enable the patient to express the reasons for seeking out a possible method for restoration of hearing.

With this nucleus of staff, the co-investigator team is ready to enter into the cooperative effort of cochlear implantation with the HEI. An extensive cochlear implant clinical trials manual is provided for each team. This contains all of the forms that are used for reporting data back to the HEI. Cochlear implant packets are received that contain questions and answers for the patients, questionnaires for them to fill out after they have read the material, and forms for collection of audiological, vestibular, radiographic, psychological, surgical and postsurgical data.

Our team functions within the confines of our private practice. We have formed a not-for-profit institute, the Midwest Ear Research Institute, to help with the postoperative evaluation and rehabilitation as we see more patients. However, the major part of our cochlear implant program is handled in clinical practice.

DESCRIPTION OF THE COCHLEAR IMPLANT

The implant system is shown in Figure 20.1. The microphone is usually attached to the side of the glass frames close to the lens. It may be worn through a shirt buttonhole, a tie clasp, or whereever the patient desires. The microphone picks up acoustic stimuli and transmits them to a stimulator unit. The signal is converted by the stimulator unit to an electrical current and transmitted to an induction coil worn externally, directly over an implanted inner coil. Magnetic induction across the skin barrier from the external to internal coil activates the electrode that has been placed through the round window into the scala tympani. Current flow is between active and ground electrodes electrically stimulating remaining auditory fibers and producing a sensation of sound.

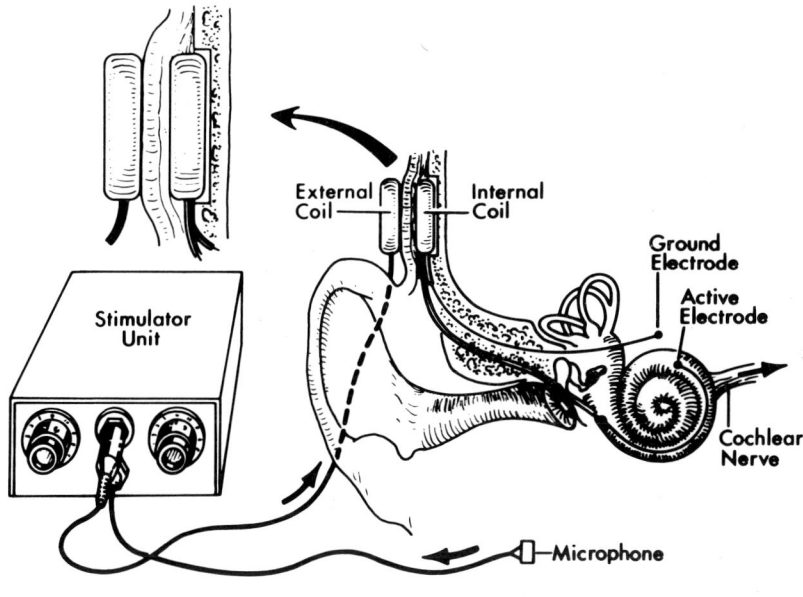

Figure 1

Cochlear Implant System

Figure 20.1. Cochlear implant system.

PATIENT SELECTION IN A CLINICAL PRACTICE

Patients are referred for consideration of a cochlear implant or they may make an appointment on their own without referral. The patient undergoes a routine audiometric evaluation and then is seen and examined by the surgeon. The patient expresses his/her desire for hearing if it could be restored. A concise explanation is given to the patient regarding the cochlear implant, its benefits, its limitations, and a booklet to read. If the patient wants to proceed with further diagnostic evaluation regarding the possibility of cochlear implantation, arrangements can be made at that time. However, in most instances, we encourage the patient to go home and read the booklet, and then we will arrange for continuation of the evaluation.

Patients may come from other geographic locations. If this is the case, we will arrange for the complete evaluation for the cochlear implant by correspondence or over the telephone. Our nurse makes arrangements for audiological testing, promontory testing (2), ENG, and polytome x-rays of the inner ear. Psychological testing is scheduled to follow these tests and requires approximately 3-4 hours of time. A cochlear implant wearer in the Kansas City area is contacted and arrangements are made for that individual to meet with the patient.

The evaluation may be fragmented into two or three parts including x-rays and promontory testing before any other extensive evaluations. In most cases, however, an orderly progression is followed beginning on a Monday morning and ending Wednesday afternoon after meeting and talking with a cochlear implant wearer. The patient is then admitted to the hospital on Thursday, sees an internist if appropriate, and undergoes surgery on Friday.

Local patients or those who have traveled to the Kansas City area relatively easily may arrive unexpectedly for evaluation for cochlear implantation. In some instances, the patient may appear to be a prospective implant candidate and did not realize it. We may fragment the evaluation and obtain basic audiometric studies, x-rays, and a promontory test. The remainder of the evaluation may be scheduled later.

Patient selection for cochlear implantation by co-investigators is based upon the following:

1. postlingually profoundly deafened individuals;
2. minimum age of 18 years;
3. psychological stability;
4. auditory nerve fibers capable of being stimulated by promontory testing; and
5. patient reliability.

Pilot programs are underway by the HEI for implantation and rehabilitation of prelingually deaf individuals. Although we perform promontory testing on all patients, strict adherance to response on promontory testing as a criteria for patient selection has not proven reliable.

AUDIOLOGICAL EVALUATION

Initial audiological evaluation of prospective candidates for the cochlear implant includes routine earphone test and impedance measurements. One change from the routine is the use of a signal light to warn the candidate when to be alert for possible presentation of a stimulus. When the light is not on, a state of vigilance is not required.

Pure tone thresholds are obtained with warble tone signals. Tape recorded spondees are utilized for attempts to obtain speech reception thresholds, however, most candidates are only able to report speech detection thresholds. It is rare that a discrimination score can be obtained from standard tests.

Subsequent tests are performed both under earphone and in the sound field. The tests include thresholds for warbled pure tones, detection of spondees, MCL, UCL, and discrimination scores for three types of word stimuli (MTS). The latter stimuli include monosyllables, trochees, and spondees. All speech stimuli are presented via tape recordings. An additional tape recorded test uses a multiple choice response procedure to determine ability to identify common environmental sounds.

When tests are performed in the sound field, a zero degree azimuth is used. Both aided and unaided conditions are evaluated. Several powerful hearing aids are tried for each ear when possible and results are compared with typical performances by cochlear implant users. The latter information is used in couseling regarding the decision to have the implant or to use hearing aids. Should the implant be elected, the information serves as baseline data for comparison to postimplant performance.

Data provided by HEI regarding average performance of typical cochlear implant patients on the MTS and environmental sounds test have been provided so that comparison can be made with these scores and the hearing aid performance of the prospective candidate.

SURGICAL SELECTION

Once it has been determined by audiometric testing that the patient most likely will benefit more by cochlear implantation than by the use of a hearing aid, perhaps the most crucial question has been answered. The other important factors include the feeling the surgeon has regarding the reliability of the patient to complete the program and cooperate to the fullest, the report of the psychologist, the input from the nurse who deals with the patient on a daily basis scheduling the tests and answering questions, and the input from the cochlear implant wearer with whom the patient has met. If the patient has a worse ear, that is the ear selected for implantation. If the patient has a preference on which ear they want operated, then that ear is selected. If the patient has no preference and both ears are the same, a decision is reached between the patient and the physician.

The surgical procedure is, briefly, as follows: A marking device is used to mark the bone above the ear before infiltration of the skin by any vasoconstrictive solution to avoid distortion of the skin. A larger than usual postauricular incision is made, well beyond the proposed seat for the implant and the avascular plane over the temporalis muscle developed.

Temporalis muscle is removed over the site for the circular seat which is then drilled into the temporal bone with a butterfly burr. A mastoidectomy is performed, a channel for the electrodes is created into the mastoid from the circular seat, and the facial recess opened. Operating through the facial recess, the bony round window lip anteriorly is removed exposing the scala tympani. Care is taken not to disturb the ossicles and not to tear the basilar membrane above the scala tympani. The inner coil is secured in its seat and the ground electrode placed so that it is against the dura in the epitympanum and its balled tip is into or close to the Eustachian tube. The active electrode is inserted through the facial recess and into the scala tympani for a distance of 18 mm. The ball tip of the electrode is at about the 3000 Hz region of the cochlea and the bare wire in the higher frequency regions. Temporalis fascia is used to seal the scala tympani, facial recess, and the postauricular incision closed. A mastoid dressing is kept in place 2 days.

The risks and complications are carefully explained to each patient and a very detailed operative permit is filled out by the patient using his/her own handwriting to write in the name of the surgeon and the operative procedure.

Patient compliance with total commitment for completing the cochlear implant program is absolutely essential. A strong intangible feeling develops between the surgeon and the patient during the evaluation. In many instances, the surgeon may feel the patient is an excellent candidate for surgery although the audiometric data may be borderline. In other instances, the audiometric data may clearly indicate a hearing aid or other device would be of no value. Regardless, this intangible feeling between the surgeon and the patient is invaluable to patient compliance and commitment to the program. The senior author cannot stress this point enough. After the patient is selected for surgery, a very special relationship develops between this patient and the surgeon.

Electronystagmography, polytomography, and plain x-rays are helpful in pre- and postoperative surgical management. For example, an individual with normal vestibular function might be advised about dizziness after surgery. Fibrosis or calcification of the cochlea on polytomography may alert the surgeon to possible difficulties inserting the active electrode into the round window and scala tympani. Plain x-rays are obtained postoperatively to check ground and active electrode placement and if the electrodes are intact.

Any medical problems the patient might have are dealt with by an internist on consultation at the time of admission to the hospital.

In paying careful attention to details preoperatively, the surgical data arrives and, generally, there are no surprises.

REHABILITATION

The External Stimulator

After cochlear implant surgery, a 2-month healing period occurs before the patient returns for fitting with the external stimulator.

The first order of business is to determine if electrical stimulation through the external coil will result in a sensation of sound. This is a very emotional moment for most patients because of the uncertainty. However, some patients are confident the device will work because they have already received stimulation from motor driven items like electric shavers, hair clippers, and garbage disposals.

Electrical signals are presented to the external coil as it is hand-held over the implanted coil. The signals originate from a threshold tester developed at HEI. The pulsed 16 KHz signal is presented at a very low voltage and a threshold is obtained in much the same way audiometric pure tone thresholds are obtained. Then the voltage is slowly increased until an uncomfortable level is determined. These measurements are obtained repeatedly until stability of response is verified.

The potentiometers of the external stimulator are set to present a signal with parameters matching the thresholds and uncomfortable levels obtained via the threshold tester. One of the potentiometers sets a carrier level agreeing with the threshold level, while the second sets a clipping level in agreement with the UCL.

The external coil is placed in a supporting device so that it will remain situated directly over the implanted internal coil. This is usually accomplished by attachment to the temples of eyeglasses. Thresholds are then retested with the threshold testing apparatus to assure maximum coil performance.

A microphone is attached to the external stimulator and voice signals are presented. Most implant recipients do not find that voices sound "normal" but rather have a "squeaky" quality. In the early stages, most cannot differentiate voices (men vs. women).

TRAINING

Training with the device is then initiated. The training program (basic guidance) follows procedures developed by Norma Norton and staff at the HEI (3). The program revolves around a nucleus of 26 hours of direct contact sessions. Additionally, a home study program is provided for the cochlear implant user. The basic guidance sessions focus on development of critical listening ability. Minimal cue training helps reinforce the multiple uses of even partial distorted speech and environmental sounds.

Sound makers are utilized to help in the determination of "same"-"different" sounds with no emphasis placed upon identification of the sound. Then differentiation of characteristics of repetitive versus steady-state sounds is emphasized. Beginning speech training materials can be differentiated or identified solely by temporal or by a combination of temporal and intensity parameters.

Besides the minimal cue training, the basic guidance program also includes speech training and monitoring of voice level and speaking rate.

Speech reading ability is evaluated through use of videotape presentations of the CHABA speech reading tests. The particular tapes used are those prepared by the National Technical Institute for the Deaf. The tests are performed very early in the basic guidance period and several times during the training period. Many conventional speech reading techniques are used and extensive auditory training without visual cues is provided.

Cochlear implant users can be taught a code to use the telephone in a limited way. The code does not allow normal conversation, but it can be used to transmit messages in both normal and emergency situations. The code, as adapted by Norma Norton from a *Speech Indicator Manual* by Ray Jones, takes advantage of an implant user's ability to differentiate a one-syllable reply from a two- or three-syllable reply. The implant user asks questions that can be answered by "yes" or "no". If the answer is no, the person talking to the implant user says no one time. If the answer is yes, the listener says yes twice. The implant user counts the number of syllables in the reply to learn the answer to the question.

DATA AND RESULTS

The etiology of deafness in the 9 patients implanted in this series was otosclerosis in 4, meningitis in 2, and acquired, unknown in three. The patients ranged in age 22–61 years at time of implant. Five were females and 4 were males. The patients had been profoundly deaf from 18 months to 25 years before implant.

In the 4 patients with otosclerosis, 2 patients had stapes surgery, 1 of which we were aware, and the other unknown. The other 2 had unoperated cochlear otosclerosis. One of these required extensive bone removal of the promontory anterior to the round window. One of the patients who had previous stapes surgery, unknown to us, also had extensive bony involvement of the promontory requiring extensive bone removal anterior to the round window niche. In all 4 patients, the active electrode was inserted the full 18 mm without difficulty. In both patients with meningitis, no extensive bone removal was required and no bony obliteration or fibrosis was present, allowing placement of the active electrode with ease. In all 3 patients who had acquired unknown postlingual deafness, there were no difficulties inserting the electrode.

Polytome x-rays in all of these patients were accurate in determining ossification of the round window and basal turn of the cochlea. The necessity of extensive bony removal of the promontory was predicted preoperatively by polytome x-ray.

Vestibular studies in these patients disclosed normal vestibular function in 2, reduced vestibular response in 2, and absent vestibular response in 5. In none of the patients did postoperative vertigo occur. Table 20.1 shows the relationship of vestibular function and etiology of deafness.

Each patient was ambulatory the morning after surgery. We chose to x-ray the patients the day after surgery for electrode placement while they were still in the hospital. In all of the patients, the active electrode placement was the full 18 mm in length. No serious kinks were present in the active electrode.

Prophylactic antibiotics are used routinely. One gram of Nafcillin is given at the time of induction of anesthesia, another gram given 4 hours later, and then discontinued. Careful attention in establishing the avascular plane overlying the temporalis fascia prevents compromising the blood flow of the postauricular skin flap. To date, no complications have occurred in our series regarding slough, extrusion, or other abnormalities of the skin flap overlying the inner coil.

One patient wears a hearing aid in one ear and the implant in the other. The most recent patient (in process) has found that a body aid in the opposite ear allows him to function at about the level a cochlear implant wearer might expect to function. We implanted his other ear with the idea that he may very well be a wearer of both implant and hearing aid.

The first 7 patients were implanted with a standard single electrode induction coil. The last 2 patients, in process, have been implanted with a coil that contains a central core magnet devised by the co-investigator team in Oklahoma City (4).

Seven patients who have been fitted with their stimulator units all wear their units on a daily basis. Warble tone mean thresholds range from 30 to 60 dB across the frequencies tested 250–3000 Hz.

The results of rehabilitation in these seven patients can be seen in Table 20.2. Comparison can be made between the performance of a typical cochlear implant wearer (Table 20.3) and the data and scores obtained from the patients undergoing rehabilitation with the cochlear implant from the Midwest Ear Research Institute. All of our patients have exceeded the low score from HEI data in environmental sounds. This includes those patients who have only had their cochlear implants during their first 2 weeks of basic guidance from which we obtained the data. The scores for MTS word recognition and MTS stress recognition can be compared. MTS words are used in a closed set. Word recognition is actual recognition of the word itself. Stress recognition is recognition of the stress placed on the syllables of the MTS words. These data compare favorably with data from the HEI and other co-investigators (5).

Table 20.1
Relationship of Vestibular Function to Etiology of Deafness

	Cochlear Implant N = 9	
Subject	Etiology	Bilateral Vestibular Function
MM	Otosclerosis	Normal
RC	Otosclerosis	Absent
DM	Meningitis	Absent
JD	Acquired, unknown	Absent
WS	Acquired, unknown	Normal
VH	Otosclerosis	RVR(R); Absent (L)
IT	Otosclerosis	RVR
DM	Meningitis	Absent
DB	Acquired, unknown	Absent

CONCLUSION

Our team functions in clinical and private practice. The basic nucleus of audiologist, psychologist, nurse, and otologist are

Table 20.2
Comparison of 7 Patients with Cochlear Implants

	Performance with a Cochlear Implant (Midwest Ear Research Institute) N = 7			
Subject	Environmental Sounds (%)	MTS Stress Recognition (%)	MTS Word Recognition (%)	Time of Test after Stimulator Fitting
MM	60	83	21	2 weeks
	75	83	42	2 years
RC	60	67	29	2 weeks
	65	67	38	2 years
DM	45	22	4	2 weeks
	50	79	25	6 months
	70	75	25	1 year
JD	60	67	25	2 weeks
	60	67	67	6 months
WS	60	62	8	2 weeks
	55	71	33	6 months
VH	70	75	25	2 weeks
IT	45	38	4	2 weeks

Table 20.3
Typical Performance with a Cochlear Implant (HEI)

	Cochlear Implant N = 45		
	Environmental Sounds (%)	MTS Stress Recognition (%)	MTS Word Recognition (%)
Low score	15	42	17
Mean score	59	81	40
High score	95	100	79

minimal. A speech pathologist and electrical engineer would offer a significant contribution to rehabilitation and further electronic alteration in the system. However, these are not absolutely essential.

Patients find the cochlear implant a continual learning experience after completion of basic guidance. Speech reading courses are strongly urged for an indefinite period once the patient returns home.

The cochlear implant is here to stay. There is no question that patients benefit from their prosthesis even though it does not allow speech discrimination as we know it. Perhaps the most important feeling our patients relate to us is a rediscovery of their own identity by hearing their own voice again.

References

1. House, W.F., Berliner, K.I., et al: Cochlear implants. *Ann Otol Rhinol Laryngol* (Suppl 27) 85: 1-92, 1976.
2. House, W.F., and Brackmann, D.E. Electrical promontory testing in differential diagnosis of sensori-neural hearing impairment. *Laryngoscope* 84: 2163-2171, 1974.
3. Norton, N.B., Eisenberg, L.S., Berliner, K.I., and Thielemeir, M.A. Cochlear implant rehabilitation manual. House Ear Institute, 1980.
4. Dormer, K.J., Richard, G., Hough, J.V.D., and Hewett, T. The cochlear implant (auditory prosthesis) utilizing rare earth magnets. *Am J Otol* 2: 22-27, 1980.
5. House, W.F., Berliner, K.I., Eisenberg, L.S., et al: The cochlear implant: 1980 update. *Acta Otolaryngol* (in press).

CHAPTER 21
Tinnitus Masking: A Critical Review

Earl R. Harford, Ph.D.

For the past 5 years, there has been increasing interest in the use of electronic devices specifically designed and built for the relief of tinnitus. These devices, called tinnitus maskers, are electronic generators, housed in hearing aid cases, that produce a band of noise intended to mask the user's tinnitus. Commercial tinnitus maskers generate broad and narrow bands of noise and have variable output controls. There are even ultrahigh frequency maskers that claim to generate signals up to 15,000 Hz. Some maskers have discrete frequency noise band adjustments, usually high, low, and midfrequency bandpass filters. There are instruments available that contain just a masking stimulus and others that consist of a hearing aid plus a masker. The former are called tinnitus maskers and the combination units are referred to as tinnitus instruments. There are about four manufacturers of tinnitus masking devices in the United States. These companies produce a total of nearly 20 different models (1).

The use of tinnitus maskers is being promoted as an effective therapeutic procedure and reports appear in newspapers and magazines about the use of tinnitus maskers and tinnitus instruments. Courses designed to train evaluators and fitters of tinnitus maskers are being held throughout the country. Although a few reports on tinnitus maskers have appeared in the professional literature, none of them are based on prospective experimental design. Most of them report clinical experience and offer descriptive data. There is still inadequate evidence in the scientific literature that maskers are a valid and viable therapeutic device for the relief of tinnitus.

The use of masking to treat tinnitus is not a new concept. An electronic device, however, that produces an acoustic stimulus especially tailored to mask a patient's tinnitus is a new concept. Ever since Vernon (2) described a clinical procedure for evaluation of tinnitus and use of masking to treat the symptom in 1976, the use of maskers has received considerable attention.

There is no standardized clinical procedure for evaluating tinnitus and for establishing a prognosis for success from a masker. In the spring of 1978, a Tinnitus Clinic was developed at the University of Minnesota Medical School to learn about tinnitus masking from first-hand experience. We have had enough positive reinforcement from our patients to continue our Clinic. Our Tinnitus Clinic has four major components:

1. the neurootologic/audiologic diagnosis,
2. the tinnitus evaluation,
3. trial use of a masking device and
4. professional follow-up counseling.

DIAGNOSIS

Tinnitus should always be considered initially as a neurotologic symptom that must be carefully evaluated to rule out a treatable disease and/or a life-threatening disorder of the central nervous system. Once the neurotological and audiological evaluation has been completed and the decision made to investigate a masker, the next step is to evaluate the tinnitus, per se. The patient may or may not have a hearing loss. If there is a hearing loss that interferes with speech communication, it is wise to investigate the use of a hearing aid before, or in lieu of, a tinnitus masker. A hearing aid *often* provides relief from tinnitus while simultaneously improving the patient's communicative efficiency. We routinely explore regular hearing aid use before a special tinnitus masking device, even if the patient has just a mild hearing loss. In the past 2 years, nearly 50% of the patients who registered in our tinnitus clinic were treated with a hearing aid to relieve their tinnitus. Recall that hearing aids have been known to offer relief from tinnitus, especially high-pitch tinnitus, for more than 40 years. The content of this paper focuses on patients with tinnitus who are not helped by, or do not warrant, a conventional hearing aid.

TINNITUS EVALUATION

A tinnitus evaluation should be conducted to establish the nature of the patient's tinnitus to determine if masking is a feasible approach and to have information for specifying the type of masking to be incorporated into a masker. Our *tinnitus evaluation* consists of five parts:

1. history,
2. pitch matching,
3. loudness matching,
4. masking, and
5. residual inhabition testing.

The first step in the tinnitus evaluation is to obtain a careful history. We are now able to use certain key questions to predict acceptance and success of a tinnitus masker by a patient. In particular, the greater the annoyance and handicap the tinnitus imposes on the patient, the more likely a tinnitus masker will be useful. Obviously, this principle applies to most prosthetic devices. Consequently, we often use our tinnitus history form as a screening mechanism for patients who write or call the clinic or come in with some other chief complaint of the ear, head or neck and subsequently learn about our Tinnitus Clinic. This history form requires that the patient think carefully about the annoyance and nature of his or her tinnitus. Some patients conclude after completing the history that their tinnitus really is not very much of a problem. We do not encourage patients to investigate tinnitus masking unless the problem has been present for a year or longer. If tinnitus persists for more than 1 year and the patient has failed to cope with it effectively, we feel that the investigation of a tinnitus masker is indicated.

The second step in our tinnitus evaluation is to present the patient with various acoustic stimuli in an effort to obtain a *pitch match*. High pitched tinnitus is most common among our patients which supports Vernon (4) and Roeser's and Price's (5) reports. Vernon states that 63% of his patients have tinnitus between 2–7 kHz. Only 21% located it below 2 kHz and 16% above 7 kHz. We agree with these figures and also find that high-pitched tinnitus (up to 8–10 kHz) is easier to mask than low-pitch tinnitus.

The third step in the evaluation is to obtain a *loudness match* of the tinnitus, using the same stimulus as that used for pitch match. The loudness of tinnitus can be misleading from the history. Even though the majority of patients report that their tinnitus is loud, most persons match loudness just a few decibels above the threshold of the stimulus that sounds like their tinnitus. Stated differently, the physical intensity of most tinnitus is not nearly as loud as the patient subjectively reports. Roeser and Price (5) report that 77% of their group of 83 patients matched the loudness of their tinnitus within a 10-dB sensation level. Our experience agrees with their report.

Tinnitus matching is easily accomplished by most patients. There are some, however, especially those with central tinnitus, who find that matching their tinnitus to an external stimulus is a very difficult or impossible task. Even though a standard clinical audiometer with variable narrow bands of noise can be used to assess the pitch and loudness of tinnitus, we have found a special tinnitus analyzer is a more effective and reliable clinical tool for evaluating the nature of tinnitus. There are tinnitus analyzers on the market now (1981).

The fourth step in the evaluation is to determine whether or not the patient's tinnitus can be masked, and if so, how much sound pressure is required to "cover" the tinnitus. There are some patients whose tinnitus cannot be masked by any signal, some are masked very easily, whereas still others experience only partial masking (mainly reduction in loudness and/or change in quality) of their tinnitus. Those with a severe hearing loss, *particularly in the frequency* range of the tinnitus, and those with central tinnitus, localized somewhere in the head, are the most difficult to mask.

The fifth step in our tinnitus evaluation is to determine whether the tinnitus disappears completely or partially after a 1-minute stimulation of the ear with a masking noise 10 dB above the minimum masking level. Vernon (4) reports that 78% of his patients claim to experience partial or complete relief from their tinnitus after a 1-minute stimulation. He refers to this phenomenon as residual inhabition. Total residual inhibition can be a very dramatic and emotional experience for a patient who has severe and constant tinnitus. Again, our experience is similar to Vernon's report.

WEARABLE TINNITUS MASKER

If the tinnitus evaluation indicates that the patient may benefit from a wearable tinnitus masker, the next logical step is to fit the patient with a device that conforms to specifications consistent with results from the tinnitus evaluation. We must meet three conditions before trying a masker:

First, the patient must be very disturbed by his tinnitus and highly motivated to obtain relief.

Second, the masking stimulus must be acceptable to the patient. That is, the stimulus used to mask the tinnitus during the evaluation should not be worse than the tinnitus itself.

Third, it was possible to partially or completely mask the patient's tinnitus during the evaluation.

When these three conditions are met, we fit the patient with a tinnitus masker that produces a noise band in the frequency range of the tinnitus. If the patient is so inclined, the fitting is followed by trial use of the masker to determine if he can learn to ignore the sound generated by the device. If passive relief, that is, residual inhibition, occurs after the masker is removed, this is an extra dividend that the patient gains from the masker. The best way to explore the use of a masker is to allow the patient to actually use such a device on a daily basis for at least 2 or 3 weeks under carefully professional surveillance and guidance. Ideally, the patient should return to the clinic at least once each week during this trial period to report his experiences and receive advice and support from the audiologist.

DISCUSSION

Degree of success with tinnitus maskers varies in the literature. I suppose a major reason is the difficulty in defining success. In a preliminary study Vernon and Scheuning (6) report that 81% of their patients were obtaining relief from tinnitus masking. Roeser and Price (5) report only 26% of their patients report help from a masker. Rose (8) reports findings similar to Roeser and Price and our experiences are also consistent with those of Roeser. According to the most current report by Vernon and his colleagues on 78 patients, those who were fitted with masking instruments report the highest degree of success. This result could be biased by improved hearing rather than relief from tinnitus. Recall that tinnitus instruments are a combination of a hearing aid and masker in the same ear.

What is not reflected by the data in published reports is the favorable effect that a Tinnitus Program or Clinic has on patients who suffer from tinnitus. The majority of our patients have been told in the past that nothing can be done for their tinnitus and that they had to learn to live with it. Many had been told that the cause is unknown. Patients are seen in our clinic for a careful neurotologic diagnosis. Those with hearing loss receive comprehensive hearing health care, some get hearing aids, some get maskers or combination aid and masker, while others get nothing. Yet the majority of our patients claim they experience emotional relief to learn that their tinnitus is not a sign of a tumor or life-threatening disease. Stated differently, a specific clinical activity that focuses on the symptom of tinnitus can do much to help patients by reducing stress from the bewilderment, anxiety, and discomfort of tinnitus. Tinnitus masking per se is not a panacea, but in my professional judgment, it has a viable role in a comprehensive hearing health care program.

There are still many questions about tinnitus maskers that have not been answered. Probably the two most significant questions are:

1. What is the long-term acceptance of tinnitus maskers by persons with tinnitus?

2. Can long-term stimulation by a tinnitus masker exascerbate tinnitus and/or cause a permanent hearing loss?

Vigorous research in months ahead should provide the answers to these and many other questions about tinnitus masking. In the meantime, we intend to continue to use masking devices with our selected patient population on a careful and systematic basis until a more effective form of management for tinnitus becomes available.

References

1. Loavenbruck, A. Tinnitus masking devices: safe and effective? *ASHA* 22: 857–861, 1980.
2. Vernon, J.A. Tinnitus. *Hearing Aid J* 13: 13, 1975.
3. Vernon, J. The loudness of tinnitus. *Hearing Speech Action*, 44: 17–19, 1976.
4. Vernon, J. American Tinnitus Association Newsletter. Vol. 3, No. 3, 1978.
5. Roeser, R.J., and Price D.R. Clinical experience with tinnitus maskers. *Ear Hearing 1:* 63–67, 1980.
6. Vernon, J., and Schleuning, A. Tinnitus: a new management. *Laryngoscope* 88: 413–419, 1978.
7. Rose, D. Tinnitus maskers: a follow-up. *Ear Hearing 1:* 69–68, 1980.

CHAPTER 22
Ménière's Syndrome and Disease

L. B. W. Jongkees, M.D.

Ménière's syndrome—the triad of cochlear and vestibular pathology together with reactions from the autonomic nervous system—has been very thoroughly examined by Dr. Prosper Ménière. He found syphilis, otitis media, trauma, intoxications, otosclerosis, diseases of the eighth nerve and many other conditions as the causes of this triad.

In some instances, these pathological conditions may lead to more or less clear attacks, but "it certainly is not all Ménière that attacks" (freely quoted from Sir Terence Cawthorne). Up to Ménière's time, the doctors believed that a cerebral congestion was the cause of the attack and prescribed a treatment in accordance with this etiological point of view but Ménière had the opportunity to examine a young patient, who died and at the postmortem examination, he found pathology in the deaf ear: a reddish substance in vestibulum and semicircular canals.

Attacks of vertigo with changes in hearing suggest Ménière's diseases but only if other diseases like syphilis, carcinosis, diabetes, ureamia, leukemia, etc., are not discovered by a thorough examination and, further, if there is no combination with loss of consciousness, headache, paralysis and if, after the attack, the patient feels well equilibrated again. In Ménière's disease, the patient is suffering from giddy spells, together with tinnitus, loss of hearing of the inner ear type, and a sensation of pressure inside and about the ear. This is usually present in people with a certain type of character—introspective, conscientious, more or less neurotic. The attacks are mostly preceded by prodromic warnings like more noise in the ear, stronger pressure, throat ache, sensations of needles and pins in a hand, and so forth. After the giddy spell, the patient usually falls asleep and, when he wakes up, the vertigo, the vomiting, the sweating, the fright have disappeared but head noises and loss of hearing may persist until the next attack. In the first stage of the disease, hearing usually fluctuates. Ménière's disese is an *idiopathic* syndrome.[1]

Dr. Ménière did not only find the combination of cochlear, vestibular and autonomous symptoms as the result of peripheral vestibular disturbances, his greatest work was the differentiation of the various diseases that could provoke the triad and the idiopathic syndrome, a real disease "sui generis" with the many specific traits which he had already described in 1861.

It may seem to be a play upon words to demand a clear differentiation between syndrome and disease coupled with the name of Dr. Ménière, but it is not, because it has very important diagnostic and therapeutic consequences. The most important being the concept of labyrinthine hydrops.[2]

As long as we are unable to differentiate between the various affections of the vestibular system that may lead to attacks of dizziness and are unsure that hydrops of the labyrinth is really and truly the regular escort of Ménière's disease and dose not accompany other affections of the inner ear like internal otitis, syphilitic disorders or is found in people in perfect health, our entire philosophy about hydrops and Ménière's disease is uncertain and probably wrong. All of the diagnostic and therapeutic inferences and actions are equally uncertain or wrong. To mix up Ménière's disease and Ménière's syndrome is turning

---

[1] Ménière's syndrome is a useful concept, not to be interchanged with Ménière's Disease, since treatment and prognosis are entirely different.
J.F. Plantenga, 1981

[2] The diagnosis of Ménière's Disease is often not justified.
W.J. Oosterveld, 1980

back medical history for more than a century.[3]

It seems likely that endolymphatic hydrops and Ménière's disease might have something in common. The former might be the cause of the latter. As long as we do not carefully separate secondary Ménière's syndrome from the idiopathic form, Ménière's disease, we shall never be able to find out what hydrops of the labyrinth means.[4]

Let us not forget that we are not yet able to diagnose endolymphatic hydrops in the living patient. Let us not forget that the first cases showing hydrops of the labyrinth were described by Hallpike and Cairns in patients suffering from Ménière's syndrome.[5]

The concept of Dr. Ménière was that apart from various kinds of secondary forms of attack with a Ménière syndrome, there is the idiopathic form, Ménière's disease. The differentiation is not always easy but it has been made unnecessarily difficult by neglecting Ménière's work. The case histories are insufficient even in famous laboratories to give the answer to the question about the correlation between endolymphatic hydrops and Ménière's disease. The greatest part of the case histories registered as Ménière's disease as the underlying disease of a histological postmortem diagnosis are either inadequate for this purpose or clearly indicate the presence of a secondary Ménière's syndrome.

But we also know that hydrops may be absent in the temporal bone of patients who have suffered from Ménière's disease (Arnvig, 1947; Brunner, 1948; Bergren, 1949; Wüstrow and Borkowsky 1960) and present in people who have never complained about dizziness (Rollin, 1940; Buchs, 1960; Sando e.a., 1976).

We shall have to explore much more extensively the labyrinth of data about Ménière, realizing that both clinical and laboratory studies are important but that only their relation can give us the final solution of the problem of Ménière.

---

[3] The name of the condition under consideration should be Ménière's disease and all other appelations included Ménière's syndrome discarded. It is not Ménière's disease but some other condition.
B. Alford, 1972

[4] In our present state of knowledge, it is clear that not only the pathogenesis but the etiology and the explanation of the functional disturbances are not yet definitely explained.
J.R. Lindsay, 1962

[5] Ménière's disease requires much more research and many more answers before we can begin properly to understand this common disease that affects so many American citizens.
H.F. Schuknecht, 1978

CHAPTER 23

Iowa Results of the Treatment of Ménière's Disease

Brian F. McCabe, M.D., and Robert T. K. Chui, M.D.

In this study, 125 patients with classic Ménière's disease were studied in depth with a view to their response to medical therapy, surgical response to endolymphatic shunt surgery, or vestibular nerve section. All patients had Ménière's disease in all aspects, with typical episodic prostrating spells of true vertigo and with unilateral (or bilateral, in 25%) deafness with all the characteristic audiometric aspects of cochlear disease.

All patients were begun with medical therapy, which consisted of a 1200 mg sodium diet, 500 mg of chlorothiazide twice daily and, in most cases, 400 mg of cyclandelate three times daily. In a small number of cases (less than 10%), diazepam is small doses (2-4 mg tid) was given for those patients with adjunctive spells of consequence to interfere with their daily life in a minor way, i.e., momentary interference with concentration, a feeling like "a severe spell was going to come but it never came off," etc. A mixture of major and adjunctive spells such as this is the rule in Ménière's disease and is almost universally elicited by the careful historian. The history of the adjunctive spell is particularly elicited from the patient who has responded to treatment for major spells.

All patients not only satisfied the AAOO ten-times rule but are 2 or more years post-treatment.

Results (n = 125)
Medical (n = 83)
 A—14%
 B—28% } 42%
 C—38%   } 75%
 D—25%

Shunt (n = 26)
 A—35%
 B—27% } 62%
 C—3%
 D—35%

Vestibular Nerve Section (n = 18)
 A—18%
 B—27% } 45%
 C—55%   (30% late drops)
 D—0

Our concept of the treatment of Ménière's disease today is that medical therapy is proper in initial stages but not solely for relief of major spells. If spells are controlled but hearing continues to disintegrate as measured either by threshold tests or discrimination scores, medical treatment must be considered a failure and surgical measures should be instituted. We favor shunt surgery as the first line of relief. It works in remarkably high number of patients, although we do not understand why. This is discussed in another chapter in this volume. Vestibular nerve section redeems all patients from major spells (if the diagnosis is correct), but saves hearing in a lesser number, suggesting that there is likely nothing in the way of a reversible role that ablative operation has to play in the way of secretomotor activity. Supportive of that concept is that one-third of our patients after vestibular nerve section who had improved or stable hearing had later significant hearing drops, presumably because the disease was still active in the cochlea.

Although the nerve section group had a smaller percentage of hearing improved or stabilized of any group, it is true that this was a doubly burdened group, having failed both medical therapy and shunting in almost every instance. Only 3 of the 125 patients had a nerve section as the primary mode of therapy and these had had medical therapy in others' hands close enough to our therapy as to not justify hope that minor changes in the program would be successful.

The results of treatment presented here are not spectacular. Other case series have been published with significantly better results. The principal reason for this difference we feel is in our definition of "control" as applied to our patients which was extremely strict. We had no category termed "improved." If a patient had a single major spell, he was considered, for the purposes of this study, a failure. This does not mean to say, however, that after one major spell he was rushed to the operating room. A patient could well be a failure in this study but quite content with his life in terms of major reduction of spells with, for example, one spell per year and stabilized hearing. In such patients, no operation was contemplated or advised. It would be easy to lump this patient into the successful group, but this temptation was avoided.

Totally destructive operations such as transcanal labyrinthotomies or transmastoid labyrinthectomy were rarely performed by us and this does not then deserve a separate treatment category. There were two reasons for the paucity of these operations. The first is that involvement of the opposite ear has to be anticipated and the younger the patient is at onset, the more likely this is to happen. The incidence of bilaterality grows over the years. Our incidence in this series was 25% but a 2-year minimum follow-up is but a short time in the natural history of a disease for which we have means of control for many but a cure for none. Bilaterality has been noted by others to be as high as 43% in multidecade follow-up. The second reason is an aversion to taking from a patient even a little hearing. Those of us working in cochlear electrode implant programs know how precious even a little hearing can be. We urge abandonment of the old "50–50" rule (50 dB SRT or less, 50% or less discrimination score) as the criterion for destructive labyrinthotomy. A destructive operation should be reserved for the patient with no hearing and uncontrolled major spells. Of the available operations, we favor the middle fossa over the translabyrinthine vestibular nerve section with preservation of the cochlear nerve (for later possible cochlear implant) because only this way can the occasional arterial loop patient be discovered and amputation neuroma of branches of the vestibular nerve be precluded.

We have made great efforts in the management of Ménière's disease in the last two decades. It is a distinct disappointment to us, however, that in spite of the energy in this direction expended by many of our colleagues and ourselves we are not a great deal closer to its control or cure than 40 years ago when the classic monograph on this condition was written by Henry "Bill" Williams, a late resident of this state.

CHAPTER 24
Treatment of Vertigo

L.B.W. Jongkees, M.D.

Because vertigo is only a symptom, it is in fact impossible to discuss treatment of vertigo. A real treatment which intends to cure is only possible if we have discovered the diagnosis of the underlying disease. In this respect, diagnosis does not merely mean the use of the word to camouflage our ignorance but insight into the pathogenesis, etiology, and the cause of ensuing functional disturbances. On the basis of this knowledge, it is often possible to treat and to cure vertigo or to predict that the complaint will either disappear spontaneously or probably will be permanent. In the latter circumstances, it may be necessary to use symptomatic measures by which to help that patient to conquer the very disagreeable situation of disturbed equilibrium.[1]

I shall not discuss the treatment of all kinds of pathology that may be the cause of giddiness: it would take hours. I shall try to say something about the smaller part of the problem because this problem represents the situation of the patient whose complaints are not provoked by a cause that we really understand: How should we treat the patient suffering from Ménière's disease?[2-9]

First of all, I want to point out that, until now, only very few authors on this subject have been able or, at least, have taken the trouble to conduct a prospective randomized trial with both treated and untreated control groups before the efficacy of a treatment was accepted. This is true for both medical and surgical forms of therapy. On top of that, hardly anybody who has published the results of treatment of patients suffering from Ménière's disease has included an adequate and appropriate follow-up. The warnings from prominent research workers in the vestibular field have not been lacking. In 1953, McNally

---

[1] As long as we do not know what Ménière's disease really is, we shall not be able to treat it. We shall be obliged to help each patient as well as we can.
[2] Paroxysmal vertigo + hearing loss and autonomic symptoms
  a. Ménière's disease
  b. Lermoyez's syndrome
  c. Labyrinthitis complicating otitis media
  d. VIIIth nerve tumours
  e. Cerebellopontine arachnoiditis
  f. Cogan's syndrome
[3] Paroxysmal vertigo (cochlear disturbances usually absent)
  a. Brain tumors
  b. Vertebrobasilar artery: ischemic disorders
  c. Cervical vertigo
[4] Very brief attacks of vertigo
  a. Childhood vertigo (vertige de l'enfant)
  b. Gerlier's disease
  c. Epileptic vertigo
  d. Migraine attacks
  e. Reflex attacks
[5] Positional or positioning vertigo
  a. Benign paroxysmal positional vertigo
  b. Positional vertigo
  c. Orthostatic vertigo
[6] Vertigo which begins abruptly and decreases slowly (with hearing impairment)
  a. Labyrinthitis
  b. Neuritis of the eighth nerve
  c. Ramsay Hunt syndrome
  d. Labyrinth trauma
[7] Vertigo which begins abruptly and decreases slowly (without hearing disorders)
  a. Vestibular neuronitis
  b. Disseminated sclerosis
  c. Cerebrovascular accident
  d. Post-traumatic vertigo of the central type
[8] Chronic vertigo with ear pathology (often changes in intensity)
  a. Chronic diseases of the ear
  b. Tumors of the eighth nerve
  c. Tuberculous meningitis
  d. Streptomycin and similar intoxications
[9] Chronic vertigo without hearing loss
  a. Syphilitic meningoencephalitis
  b. Syringobulbia
  c. Cerebral vertigo of elderly people
  d. Disseminated disorders of the brain
  e. Fainting fits, sometimes described as dizziness
  f. Hyperventilation syndrome

(1) exclaimed: "Ménière's disease, a 5-year recovery is necessary before the results of treatment can be judged." Torok (2) stated about the treatment of Ménière's disease: "A bewildering number of concepts and methods have been suggested as the best answers until the next claim of success shatters the popularity of earlier allegations."[10,11]

Let us admit that we do not know exactly what Ménière's disease is, let us accept that there is not one treatment of patients who suffer from this capricious, fickle, unpredictable disease that has been proved to have more success than some kind words, some sort of regime, or some other suggestive therapy. Whatever we do, from psychotherapy to surgery, gives us a more or less constant result of about 80% success and 20% failure (2). The only important thing is that the doctor believes in the treatment he uses. After a study of the literature on the medical treatment of Ménière's disease in 187 articles discussing this subject, I stated that I had to admit being very sad about the low standard of the greatest majority of those papers (3). Only three papers, all of them about antihistaminics, gave the positive results of a prospective, double blind, controlled study. Many of the papers were written about treatments that were based on the faith of the author in some theory, usually about the cause of hydrops of the labyrinth: disturbed water or salt metabolism, allergy, vitamine deficiencies, but also about tonus difference in the centers of the eye muscles, wrong position of vertebrae, etc.[12]

The diversity of theories, hypotheses, and statements about the nature of Ménière's disease is, in itself, quite harmless and even useful if it leads to investigations to either prove or disprove the validity of the conception.

As soon as the same theories are applied to a patient who has been diagnosed as suffering from Ménière's disease, however, they do not remain harmless because they so often lead to aggressive and unpleasant therapies.

Many a doctor often is lured into submitting his patients to all manner of disagreeable treatments (salt-free diet, endless antiallergic treatments, fluid restriction, prohibition of alcohol, sugar, smoking, etc.) or surgical therapy, based on theoretical views that are not sufficiently substantiated. Besides, I have seen too many patients healed by methods intended to cure hydrops of the labyrinth who, in fact, were suffering from something quite different.

Usually, the good success of the treatment was proved in groups of fewer than 10 patients followed for less than 3 months. It seems incredible but in the 16 years since then, not much has been changed. Yet the drugs we use are different as is the recommended therapy or surgery. In the case of surgery upon the endolymphatic sac, Torok's 80% is found again and it does not really matter at all whether one only decompresses the sac, incises it, drains it, or puts muscle flaps upon it. I cannot prove, but I feel rather sure that not finding the sac has no influence either on the results. Let us not forget that the now almost abolished labyrinthectomy usually left the patient deaf with tinnitus and motor instability. But hardly anybody published this part of the truth. After Bretlau's thorough experiment had been published, proving that the operations upon the sac are not more than placebo operations, the number of operations upon the endolymphatic sac does not seem to have diminished very much, if at all. Endolymphatic sac surgery was started on the basis of a theory. The results should have been very carefully assessed, especially because nobody has ever found a hydrops of the endolymphatic sac. It has not been done! The love for action in surgeons seems to be stronger than the love

---

[10] A 5 year recovery is necessary before the results of treatment can be judged.
W.J. McNally, 1953

[11] A bewildering number of concepts and methods have been suggested as the best answers until the next claim of success shatters the popularity of earlier allegations.
N. Torok, 1977

[12] If we want to judge the effect of a drug in a case of Ménière's disease, we must undertake a prospective double blind investigation between the drug and a placebo.

of knowledge. They prefer to go on doing operations that have a great chance of success: 80% is not such a bad result, but it is the same as that of some kind words and attention, some innocent drugs like antihistaminics, or some body exercise. The danger of the latter treatment is less and so are the action and the glory. The man with the knife is "in" today. Let him be careful not to operate only because surgery is possible.[13]

Vertigo causes fright. Any vertigo! This makes many of those patients averse to move about; they tend to remain seated or even to stay in bed though the best way to behave is to walk as much as possible, the only way to regain normal stability again is by adaptation, i.e., by training and by exercise—careful exercise, of course.

Because I am speaking to otologists, I think I should limit myself to the discussion of vestibular vertigo, but the general rules about understanding the patients' psychic problems, stimulating them to body exercise and of trying to find the underlying disease remain the same in both vestibular and nonvestibular cases. Treatment of the causal disease is of primary importance but not always possible or effective. Even if the cause of the giddiness has a name its pathogenesis may be unknown (like in Ménière's disease).

I am sure that treatment of these patients should commence from this point, i.e., their fright must be taken away by giving them confidence in their doctor. The doctor who is sure about himself and about the treatment he is giving the patient will have the best chance to make his patient trust him. This is the reason why some doctors use treatments with striking success which have no results in the hands of others. The use of prismatic spectacles is, I think, a typical example. Those who really believe in this treatment cure their patient, those who do not share their faith, have no success.

The fact that this strong psychic influence is present proves that there are circumstances, dependent upon the psychical condition of the patient, which are of the greatest importance for the possibility to cure the sufferers from Ménière's disease.

I am afraid that I myself am an incurable disbeliever as regards many theories about the origin of Ménière's disease. I am not convinced that hydrops labyrinthi depend upon disturbed water or salt metabolism, allergy, tonus differences in the centers of the eye muscles, or so many other things brought forward by those who "successfully" treat these patients according to their theory. As so many psychic influences seem to find their way towards somatic deviations via the condition of the vessels, I may follow those who try to influence Ménière's disease by provoking hyperemia, either locally or generally.

Personally, I think the first step in treating a patient, suffering from Ménière's syndrome is the examination. The doctor has to show the patient that he is interested. The anamnesis has to be very thorough, not only to exclude all other ailments which may cause spells of vertigo, but also to show the patient that his complaints are taken very seriously, that (s)he is taken seriously. Too often the doctor hears the word vertigo and has his prescription ready without giving the patient the opportunity to free his/her soul from the many things which oppress him/her. It is inadmissable not to examine the patient very thoroughly because this is the only way to really gain his/her confidence, the basis for all treatment. I remember quite well the many patients who, after a thorough examination in the torture chamber of the vestibular department told me that they felt much better already since we had been able to cause in them, artificially, sensations equal to those they felt during an attack of vertigo. Many others have surely had the same experience.

This is the point from which to start treatment. First of all, the patient should be brought back to normal life as much as possible. A great many of our patients, having a sedentary life already, eating, smoking, and drinking too much already, having too little bodily exercise, and living

---

[13] If the editors would decide not to accept any paper that does not fulfill at least one of two reasonable demands—double blind (or at least matched control groups) and a follow-up of at least 5 years—the standing of our journals would rise.

under too great a strain already, only get worse as soon as the vertigo attacks start. They hardly dare to go out, grow fatter, smoke and drink more, and live under a greater strain as a result of the psychic condition brought about by their complaints.

The patient must be brought to return to a normal life often a life much more normal than the one (s)he lived before the first signs of his trouble began to show. (S)he should be induced to take bodily exercise—walking, swimming, playing golf, or all such sports that have no element of personal competition in it. (S)he should eat lots of vegetables and fruit and take care lest (s)he grows too fat. Smoking and drinking should not be excessive. A holiday away from work, household, or other responsibilities or strain is of paramount importance to start a successful treatment, at least if the patient can abstain from the modern way of spending holidays by consuming miles, climbing mountains, or such things and in that way nearly killing her/himself, so that (s)he can only save his/her life by quickly returning to routine work. For those who can afford it a sea voyage sometimes works miracles. Surely the doctor should take care that this patient sleeps well. If necessary (s)he should not be too reluctant in giving soporifics. It may also be necessary to help that patient fight his nervous tension by giving him sedatives. I must confess I prefer the older type: bromine salts, valerian, and such to the new drugs which are so effective in various other respects.

If the treatment of the Ménière patient starts with those general measures, it is possible to spare the patient and the doctor a great many disappointments. In many cases, these measures will be enough to eliminate the patient's troubles and, in many other cases, a treatment that is thought to be directed against the pathological condition of the inner ear will have a much better chance.

I feel sure that many ways lead to success provided the doctor believes in them and is able to make the patient believe in them. It is of no importance whether the treatment is medical or surgical.

References

1. McNally, W.J. Some remarks about dizziness—its diagnostic significance and treatment. Ann Otol 62: 607–630, 1953.
2. Torok, N. Old and new in Meñière's disease. Laryngoscope 87: 1870–1877, 1977.
3. Jongkees, L.B.W. Medical treatment of vertigo. Proceedings of the Eighth International Congress of Otorhinolaryngology, Tokyo, 1965.
4. Bretlau, P. Endolymphatic sac decompression compared to a sham decompression. Shambaugh Workshop 6, Chicago, 1980.

CHAPTER 25

Critical Review of Endolymphatic Ear Surgery

Michael M. Paparella, M.D.

The author's experience and initial skepticism regarding endolymphatic sac surgery for intractable Ménière's disease are discussed against the perspective of other methods of sac surgery described in the literature. This experience encompasses 15 years. Evolution of the current method of coping with the morphological vagaries of Trautmann's triangle in the performance of sac enhancement surgery are discussed. After reviewing and discussing results, pathophysiological considerations of the role of endolymph in Ménière's disease and in patients receiving sac enhancement procedures are considered.

Any disease of unknown pathogenesis which produces incapacitating symptoms provides a field day for so-called "experts" to develop and expound theories and treatment methodologies. Such a dramatic disease is Ménière's disease.

Although art in medicine and Ménière's disease by far exceeds science, the patient with this disturbing and progressive disease desperately needs help. It is the otologist's responsibility to assist the patient with whatever tools and knowledge are at his disposal. It is the intent of therapy to ameliorate symptoms and findings conservatively, especially vertigo, with the additional objectives of preserving function and arresting the progressive nature of the disease process.

Conservative treatment of Ménière's disease is stressed using medical and psychological support mechanisms. Surgery, namely endolymphatic sac enhancement, is considered only in long-term patients who have reached a state of intractability. My purpose is not to defend sac surgery but, rather, to recount and review my experience in treating Ménière's disease over the past 14 years. I understand skeptics of this procedure as I too was very skeptical in the beginning while I sporadically used the method and chose not to discuss it at meetings during that time. Subsequently, as experience, reliable application of the method, and opportunity to objectively assess long-term results evolved, I became convinced that the method works for most patients, especially for vertigo.

MEDICAL CONSIDERATIONS

The diagnosis of Ménière's disease is largely made from the history. History is based on the following items in decreasing priority of importance:

1. Vertigo
2. Hearing loss
3. Pressure
4. Tinnitus
5. Loudness intolerance
6. Displacusis
7. Family history
8. Stress
9. Previous treatment

Of these, vertigo, hearing loss, and pressure seem most important. Because such patients have a high anxiety apprehension titer, they are strongly advised to answer the questions briefly and succinctly. Ancillary tests, especially audiometry and ENG, are essential. The early low tone loss leading to a flat audiometric lesion in Ménière's disease is well known. In many patients, we noted a peak audiometric pattern with comparatively good hearing at 2000 CPS, with poorer hearing below and above that point to be a common configuration. The patient is treated conservatively for a long and indefinite period of time using all of the various empirical methods of management. In our opinion, the most important aspect of conservative treatment is psychological assurance used pre- and postoperatively. Other diagnoses are ruled out. Glycerol tests are done routinely, although they have not demonstrated predictive significance in these cases.

UNILATERAL VS. BILATERAL

When advocating a therapeutic approach to Ménière's disease, a serious consideration is the possibility of bilateral or possible long-term involvement of the second ear in patients considered to have unilateral disease. In the literature, the incidence of bilateral involvement varies from 2-78%, obviously indicating the true incidence to be somewhere in between.

With Dr. Matt Griebe's assistance, we recently reviewed 294 patients with the definite clinical picture of Ménière's disease and found clear-cut evidence of bilaterality in 16.3% of the patients. Along with other symptoms and findings, the audiometric configuration was of special interest. Early Ménière's disease is generally described as being associated with a low frequency audiometric loss while advanced Ménière's disease is usually identified with a flat audiometric pattern. However, in our study, a "peak" audiometric configuration with better hearing at 2000 CPS and poorer hearing below and above that frequency was commonly found. Of the 342 ears with clinical Ménière's disease, 218 or 63.7% exhibited some evidence of a peak audiogram.

The time course of when the second ear became involved also was studied in patients with bilateral disease. The onset of bilateral involvement within 2 years after involvement of the first ear was experienced by 55.6%, 29.6% had symptoms 3-5 years later, and 14.8% had involvement after a period of 5 years or more, the longest being 15 years.

INCIPIENT MÉNIÈRE'S DISEASE

In addition, because peak audiograms where a low tone rises at 2000 CPS and then falls again were seen so often, they were classified and grouped according to the following criteria:

Type I: Less than 15 db loss with a gradual peak.

Type II: Sharp rise, usually to 2000 Hz, then sharp fall.

Type III: Flat, moderate to severe sensorineural hearing loss with evidence of rise, again usually at 2 kHz with subsequent fall-off.

It is beyond the scope of this chapter to hypothesize the physiology of hydrodynamics which might account for an explanation of the peak audiometric finding.

The possibility of incipient Ménière's disease in the noninvolved side should be considered. After subtracting those patients with definite Ménière's disease, 234 of 246 patients demonstrated some slight or greater abnormality on pure tone audiometry in the contralateral ear. This high incidence is in general agreement with an earlier study by Jongkees (1). Although many extrinsic and intrinsic etiological factors could be cited to explain these abnormalities, an important question remains. How many of these so-called normal ears might have incipient Ménière's disease? Could the peak audiometric configuration be of predictive value in those cases? Of these patients, 23.6% exhibited a peak pattern in the other ear; most were type I, but a few were type II. If it is valid to add this number to those with definite Ménière's disease in the second ear, we could then conclude that 30% or more patients with Ménière's disease have, or could have, Ménière's disease in the second ear. To extend this concept farther, if other kinds of hearing losses in the opposite ear are a possible indication of bilateral disease of incipient Ménière's, then theoretically, up to 30% of patients could have bilateral Ménière's disease. A study comparing the hearing of the opposite ear in unilateral Ménière's disease with normals according to age would be of interest. To follow-up on this logically, if one-third or more of these patients have Ménière's disease in the opposite ear, then clearly this supports the contention for a conservative approach on the first ear; first medically and then surgically if necessary.

PATHOPHYSIOLOGICAL CONSIDERATIONS

Whether one accepts the longitudinal or radial flow theory of endolymph or both theories, it is generally understood that endolymphatic hydrops is likely due to an excess of endolymph production or a deficiency of endolymph absorption. The stria vascularis is considered the prime site for endolymph production, while the endolymphatic sac is believed to be the most important site for endolymph absorption. Assuming endolymphatic hydrops to be a significant pathological correlate for Ménière's disease, any procedure which improves endolymph absorption should lead to a long-term lessening of hydrops and an improvement of symptoms or findings. This is true whether due to excessive production, deficient absorption, or both.

Most patients with Ménière's disease have symptoms and findings of both the cochlear and vestibular labyrinth. However, we have observed that a significant number of patients will present a clinical picture of vestibular Ménière's disease with episodic and unrelenting vertigo, pressure, and a hypovestibular caloric response to stimulation in the absence of cochlear findings of hearing loss or tinnitus. Conversely, occasional patients demonstrate pressure, fluctuating hearing, and tinnitus in the absence of vestibular findings and symptoms. Often these patients with partial labyrinthine involvement will ultimately develop the full-blown picture of Ménière's disease. To date, our experience indicates that patients with intractable vestibular Ménière's disease have more superior results than patients with full-blown clinical or cochlear Ménière's disease following sac enhancement procedures. The role of the utriculoendolymphatic valve in limiting hydrops in the vestibular versus cochlear partition in these variants of Ménière's disease is hypothesized.

SURGICAL RATIONALE

Destructive surgery for Ménière's disease includes either otological procedures (partial or complete labyrinthectomy) or intracranial procedures (vestibular neurectomy). Obviously, destructive procedures destroy and are not expected to retain or improve function. Moreover, destructive procedures are associated with increased morbidity and complications. We are all familiar with the stormy recovery period or the long-term positional dizziness a postlabyrinthectomy patient experiences. Also, most otoneurologists who advocate vestibular neurectomy as the first surgical treatment of choice have noted occasional serious complications including, in rare instances, death. Surely, if I were a patient with disturbing vertigo and intractable Ménière's disease, I would prefer a procedure which would help preserve and, hopefully, improve labyrinthine function while reducing risk and morbidity. Also, I would select an ear operation as compared to a brain operation for similarly obvious reasons. The goal of endolymphatic sac surgery is to continue conservation and preservation of function by enhancing absorption of endolymph while reducing risk.

METHOD

The primary goal is to enhance endolymph absorption function. The steps which are designed to help achieve this function include the following possibilities:

1. Enlargement of the sac;
2. Releasing bony pressure on the sac;
3. Providing intralumental surfaces of silastic along which nanoliters of endolymph can diffuse;
4. Providing collateral blood supply;
5. Use of gold foil to prevent fibroblastic postoperative sac invasion.

The specific steps of the method currently employed are as follows:

1. A complete simple mastoidectomy using a postauricular approach thinning the posterior bony canal wall, enlarging the aditus, and identification of the incus.
2. Drilling of the solid angle, but *never* below the level of the dome of the horizontal semicircular canal.
3. Thinning of bone over Trautmann's triangle and lateral sinus.
4. Using a fenestrometer, 10 mm is meas-

ured from the tip of the short process of the incus or fossa incudis along the axis of the horizontal semicircular canal (30° from the tegmen) and a point is mentally marked; then 12 mm is measured from the fossa incudis at an angle of 45° from the tegmen as it includes the posterior inferior semicircular canal which must be avoided.

5. The dura is uncovered by removing bone around the zone, and in an exaggerated way in the infralabyrinthine cell tract or region as the sac is commonly found inferior and anterior to the tip of the posterior semicircular canal.
6. If there is no Trautmann's triangle, the lateral sinus is decompressed and retracted downward to gain access below the posterior semicircular canal.
7. The sac is entered beneath the solid bony shelf by depressing the dura, opening the sac with a sickle knife, and bluntly probing the sac lumen to see the shiny epithelial lining. An inserted whirly bird can usually be twirled gently within the sac.
8. Silastic sheeting (0.005 inches) is cut in "T"-shape struts and is coiled within the sac with a stem entering into the mastoid. Spacers are used to separate the dura from the bone of the posterior canal.
9. Gelfoam moistened with an antibiotic steroid solution is placed on top.
10. Gold foil is then applied over the gelfoam to prevent postoperative fibroblastic invasion of the sac. A fascial graft is placed on top and held with additional gelfoam. A myringotomy tube is usually placed in the tympanic membrane to assist postoperative healing unless the subarachnoid space is uncovered (a rare occurrence).
11. Meticulous attention must be paid to remove bone dust, debris, etc., from the wound to avoid postoperative wound infection which can quickly spread to labyrinthitis.

The most important surgical pitfall is nonentry of the sac lumen. I am convinced that in my earlier cases, the lumen was not bluntly probed and the shining epithelium seen. It is easy to create a false lumen in the fibrous dura. Another pitfall to be avoided is inadvertently entering the posterior semicircular canal. Both exposure of the sac in the infralabyrinthine cell tract which leads to the jugular bulb region and our method of measurement helps avoid the above pitfalls. Other pitfalls include bleeding from the lateral sinus (treated by pressure and gelfoam), exposure of spinal fluid and postoperative wound infection, all of which should be controllable.

RESULTS

Results from sac surgery must be considered soft data, as contrasted with destructive procedures, such as labyrinthectomy or vestibular neurectomy, where results could be considered more definitive. This is because with sac surgery, the underlying disease continues although symptoms and findings often improve because of presumed enhancement of endolymph absorption. Several patients with frequent daily or weekly episodes of vertigo have been observed over a period of years. In these patients, vertigo was eliminated only to recur with less frequency, for example, 3 years after surgery. Moreover, the indications for surgery and the many variables of both Ménière's disease and syndrome will profoundly influence any reported results.

We used, and agree with, the variations of Ménière's described in the AAOO Committee Report which includes both vestibular and cochlear Ménière's disease. The current study includes 176 cases since our last report. Of these patients, 155 were considered to have Ménière's disease while 21 of these cases had Ménière's syndrome with known causes. A listing of this latter group includes:

1. chronic or recurrent otitis media in Ménière's syndrome;
2. delayed hydrops;
3. otosclerosis and Ménière's syndrome;
4. post-traumatic hydrops;
5. Lues and Ménière's syndrome.

The results as seen in the Ménière's disease group are summarized in Table 25.1. It is of interest that 10 patients who developed Ménière's disease in childhood are included in the classical Ménière's disease group.

The duration of Ménière's disease in this group before surgery ranges from 1-26 years with an average duration of 6.8 years. This addresses our philosophy of interceding in Ménière's disease only after it has reached a refractory state after prolonged conservative therapy. The patients

Table 25.1
Symptoms on which Diagnosis of Ménière's disease is made

1. Vertigo
2. Hearing Loss
3. Pressure
4. Tinnitus
5. Loudness intolerance
6. Diplacusis
7. Family history
8. Stress
9. Previous Rx

ages were from 9-80 years of age with the average being 46 years. Follow-up ranged between 1 year, as of this writing, to 98 months with an average of 40.5 months.

It is also of interest that 5 patients had Ménière's disease in their only hearing ear. In each case, the opposite labyrinth was functionless due to another disease process earlier in the patient's lifetime. In each instance, surgery was considered only when the hearing dropped to moderate or severe levels with prolonged and incapacitating vertigo. These cases are of special interest because of the elimination of influence from the opposite side. In each of these cases, vertigo was eliminated and hearing improved. These cases, as was true of vestibular Ménière's disease, turned out to have the best results in that vertigo was eliminated while hearing, pressure, and tinnitus were also improved in most instances.

DISCUSSION

Recently, articles by Bretlau and Thomsen et al. (2) using a double blind, placebo-controlled study on endolymphatic sac shunt surgery, have been described in the literature. I asked Dr. Chap Le, a biostatistician and member of the faculty of the School of Public Health of the University of Minnesota, for his review and opinion. Although he found no fault with the double blind design of the study, and here I refer to a recent article in the *Archives of Otolaryngology*, he "still could not believe the authors conclusions. For example, the analysis of Total Score—Figure 2, gives the impression that the treatment group is much more effective and, in the placebo group there is no difference between the preoperative versus postoperative scores. But the author's conclusions are in the opposite direction (page 272, 2nd paragraph of Results)." Further, I might observe patient selection or entry criteria included only 6 months of duration of disease and we all recognize the changeable nature of Ménière's disease. Our patients described here had an average disease duration of 6.8 years and in no instance was surgery considered so soon after the onset of Ménière's disease. The Danish study included small numbers; 15 patients with Ménière's disease and some patients had bilateral disease. The surgery was performed at two different hospitals by different people without any detailed knowledge of surgical technique or whether, for example, the lumen was identified appropriately in each case—all providing more variables to try to control. In otology, stapedectomy and tympanoplasty are established procedures and without, to my knowledge, any double blind studies having been applied. Each patient serves as his own best control. Statistics and surgery both represent important tools which should be applied appropriately and like compared to like. To paraphrase a cogent statement once made: "many a sound idea has suffered or died at the alter or pseudoalter of statistics."

References

1. Jongkees, L. Treatment of vertigo. Presented at the Third Annual International Symposium on Clinical Otology, September 3-5, 1981.
2. Thomsen, J., Bretlau, P., Tos, M., and Johnsen, N. Placebo effect in surgery for Ménière's disease. *Arch Otolaryngol* 107: 271-277, 1981.

Index

ABR: see Auditory brainstem response
Acoustic tumors, variable clinical presentations, 91–100
ACTH, sudden hearing loss and, 131
Adenoidectomy
　Children's Hospital of Pittsburgh study, 24
　eustachian tube function and, 25–30
　treatment of otitis media, 21
Adrenocorticotropic hormone: see ACTH
Aerodynamic implosive fistula mechanisms, 121
Allograft
　incus, 53
　malleus, 53, 56
Allograft ossiculoplasty
　autogenous incus remodeling, 52
　prefabricated, 52, 59–67
　　special problems, 56
　surgical techniques, 54
Antimicrobial therapy, otitis media and, 5
Atelactasis, tympanic membrane-middle ear, 9
Auditory brainstem response (middle latency), 114–117
Auditory brainstem response (short latency), 105
　abnormal, disorders associated with, 112
　anatomical origins, 106
　clinical applications, 109
　limitations, 112
　response parameters, 107
　stimuli, 106
Autogenous incus remodeling, 52
Autoimmune inner ear disease, 137, 138

Bone "rivet" columella, 54
Bony closure, stapedectomy failure and, 86
Branhamella catarrhalis, otitis media and, 5

Chemoprophylaxis, recurrent acute otitis media with effusion, 7
Children's Hospital of Pittsburgh, study of tonsillectomy and adenoidectomy, 24
Cholesteatoma, 10
　postoperative late hearing results, 41
　recurrence of, 39
　residual
　　definition, 68
　　planned revision, 71
　　surgical philosophy, 68
　　unplanned revision, 71
　surgery with obliteration, 38
　surgical methods for removal, 39
Chorda-tensor fold, 46
Cochlear implantation, single electrode, 139–146
Collagen, 36
　degradation, 37
Columella: see Long columella; Short columella

Diphtheroids, chronic otitis media and, 9
Drum, reinforcement of, cartilage for reconstruction of, 45

Ear canal
　retraction pockets, 48
　size after obliteration, 39
Endolymphatic hydrops, sudden hearing loss and, 129
Epitympanectomy, 45
Escherichia coli, chronic otitis media and, 9
Eustachian tube
　axis, 49
　function, adenoidectomy and, 25–30
　middle ear, 11
　　dysfunction, 12, 13
　　inflation, 11
　tympanoplasty, 45

Fixed footplate, stapedectomy failure and, 87

Gelfoam, revision stapedectomy, 87, 89
Golf-tee columella: see Short columella

Heamophilus influenzae, otitis media and, 5, 8, 9
Heparin, sudden hearing loss and, 131
Hydrodynamic explosive fistula mechanisms, CSF system, 120
Hypotympanum, 119

Incus allograft, 54
Incus bypass procedures
　hearing results, 88
　indications, 88
Incus necrosis, stapedectomy failure and, 86
Infection, sudden hearing loss and, 128

Labyrinthine fistulas
　acoustic/blast trauma, 122
　blunt ear trauma, 121
　congenital, 118
　explosive routes, 124
　flying and diving barotrauma, 122
　head trauma, 121
　implosive routes, 124, 125
　penetrating ear trauma, 122
　surgical aspects of repair, 123
　traumatic, 120
　tubotympanic compression, 122
Long columella, 54, 57

Malleal trough, 55
　technique, allograft, 54
Malleus allograft, 53
Malleus head, 48
Mastoid cavity
　open, diseased, 73
　　management of, 74
　surgery, 73, 75
Medial attic wall
　atrophic, reconstruction, 47
　cartilage for reconstruction of, 45
Meniere's disease, 151, 152
　Iowa results of treatment of, 153
　sudden hearing loss and, 129

Index

Micrococci, chronic otitis media and, 9
Middle cranial fossa surgery, 101–103
Middle ear
  cleft, ventilation routes in, 46
  eustachian tube, 11–13
  high negative pressure, 9

Obliterative otosclerosis, revision stapedectomy, 87, 89
Ossicular reconstruction
  hearing after surgery, 43
  total, 45
    results, 50, 51
Ossicular tissue, 48
Otitis media
  acute with effusion, 3
  adenoidectomy and, 21
  bacteriology, 5
  chemoprophylaxis for 7
  chronic with effusion, 7
  complications and sequelae, 14
  epidemiology, 3
  methods of therapy, 2
  pathogenesis, 1
  recurrent, 7
  tonsillectomy and, 21
  tympanostomy tube therapy for, 17
Otosclerosis surgery fistulas, 119
Oval window fistula, stapedectomy and, 86

Perichondrium, 54
Perilymph fistulas, sudden hearing loss and, 122
Politzer method, 11
Preoperative dead ears, revision stapedectomy, 87
Prosthesis
  displaced, stapedectomy failure and, 86
  short, stapedectomy failure and, 86
Purulent otorrhea, tonsillectomy and adenoidectomy, 22

Retraction pockets, 48
  postoperative
    avoidance, 69, 70
    definition, 68
    development, 69
    prevention, 70
    surgical philosophy, 68, 69
    treatment, 70
Rod columella: see Long columella

Sensorineural hearing loss, following stapedotomy, 80
Sensorineural impairment, revision stapedectomy, 88
Septal cartilage, 47
Short columella, 53, 58
Silastic sheeting, 47–49
Single electrode cochlear implantation, 139–146
Stapedectomy
  causes of failure, 86
  primary, 85
  revision
    dead ears as a result of, 88
    experiences with, 85
    guidelines for, 90
    hazards of, 89
    inner ear symptoms, 89
    miscellaneous comments, 88
    preoperative dead ears, 87
    preoperative hearing impairment, 87
  vs. stapedotomy, 78–83
Stapedotomy
  sensorineural hearing loss following, 80
  technique of, 80, 81
  vs. stapedectomy, 78–83
Staphylococcus aureus, otitis media and, 5, 8, 9
α-Streptococci, chronic otitis media and, 9
Streptococcus pneumoniae, otitis media and, 5, 8, 9
Streptococcus pyogenes, otitis media and, 5, 8
Sudden hearing loss
  ACTH and, 131
  heparin and, 131
  infection, 128
  Meniere's disease, 129
  metabolic, 129
  postoperatively, 129
  traumatic, 128
  tumor formation, 128
  vascular, 130
Superior malleolar fold, 46
Superior malleolar ligament, 46
Systematic epitympanectomy, 48

Temporal bone necrosis fistulas, 118
Temporalis fascia, 47
Tinnitus masking
  diagnosis, 147
  evaluation, 148
  wearable masker, 149
Tonsillectomy
  Children's Hospital of Pittsburgh study, 24
  treatment of otitis media, 21
TORP's, 49–51
  columella type, 50
Transmastoid drainage, 46, 47
Trauma, sudden hearing loss and, 128
Tumor formation, sudden hearing loss and, 128
Tympanic membrane, prefabricated allograft ossiculoplasty, 59–67
Tympanoplasty
  goals of, 45
  postoperative retraction pockets and residual cholesteatoma, 68
  staging, 48
Tympanosclerosis
  cause and prevention of, 31
  clinical, 36
  experimental, 33
  pathogenesis of, 33
Tympanostomy tube therapy
  otitis media, 17
    potential benefits, 18
    potential disadvantages, 17

Valsalva method, 11
Ventilation routes, middle ear cleft, 46